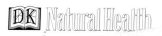

DK Natural Health

Se

REFLEX

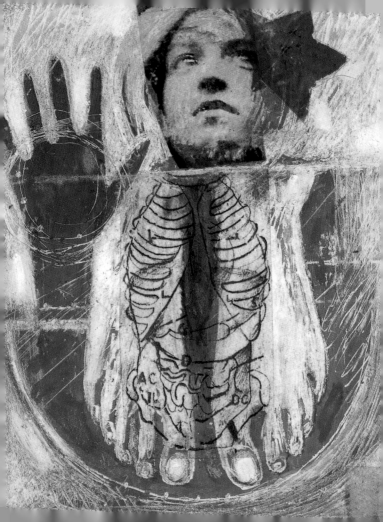

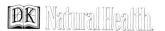

Natural Health.

Secrets of

REFLEXOLOGY

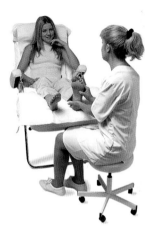

CHRIS MCLAUGHLIN
AND NICOLA HALL

A Dorling Kindersley Book

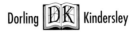

Dorling DK Kindersley

LONDON, NEW YORK, MUNICH,
MELBOURNE, and DELHI

This book was conceived, designed, and produced by
THE IVY PRESS LIMITED,
The Old Candlemakers, Lewes, East Sussex BN7 2NZ

Art director *Peter Bridgewater*
Editorial director *Sophie Collins*
Designers *Kevin Knight, Siân Keogh*
Editors *Sara Harper, Mandy Greenfield, Rowan Davies*
Picture researcher *Liz Eddison*
Photography *David Jordan*
Illustrations *Mike Courtney, Ivan Hissey, Anna Hunter-Downing,
Lesley Ann Hutchings, Andrew Milne, Sarah Young*
Three-dimensional models *Mark Jamieson*

First published in The United States of America in 2000 by
DK PUBLISHING INC,
375 Hudson Street, New York, NY, 10014
Reprinted 2002

Natural Health ® is a registered trademark of Weider
Publications, Inc. *Natural Health* magazine is the
leading publication in the field of natural self-care. For
subscription information call 800–526–8440 or visit
www.naturalhealthmag.com

Copyright © 2000 The Ivy Press Limited

A CIP catalog record for this book is available
from the US Library of Congress.

ISBN 0-7894-6778-X

Originated and printed by
Hong Kong Graphics and Printing Limited, China

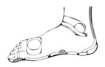

see our complete product line at

www.dk.com

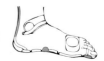

CONTENTS

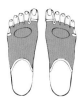 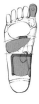 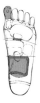

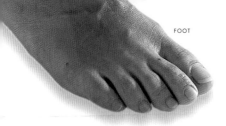

FOOT

HOW TO USE THIS BOOK

To make *Secrets of Reflexology* user-friendly, it has been divided into distinct sections, starting with one on the basic principles of reflexology (including maps of the hands and feet), and moving onto details of what happens during a treatment session. This is followed by separate sections describing how to work on all the reflex points of the hands and feet. For information on how to treat a particular reflex turn to the fifth section, "Reflexology for Healing," which forms the core of this book. The final section covers reflexology for special cases, such as babies and children, pregnant women, and older people.

Important Notice

If you have a high temperature, deep-vein thrombosis, phlebitis, a high-risk pregnancy, or severe osteoporosis, you should not receive reflexology treatment. It is also important to inform your doctor or complementary therapist that you are undergoing reflexology, in case it interferes with any prescribed medication or complementary treatments.

Do not use reflexology to replace medical treatment you are receiving for any severe problems.

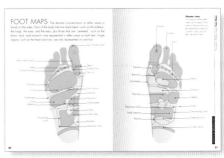

Principles

This section describes the background to reflexology and includes hand and foot maps.

Basics

This section explains what happens during a treatment session.

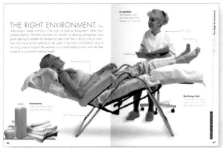

THE RIGHT ENVIRONMENT

A foot session

Here, the different reflex areas of the foot are shown in turn, photographically and in diagrams, for ease of identification.

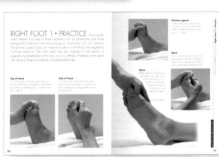

RIGHT FOOT 1 • PRACTICE

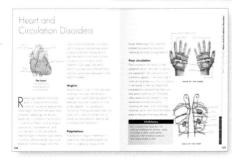

Heart and Circulation Disorders

Healing

In this section specific reflex areas are covered in detail, in terms of both theory and practice.

Introduction

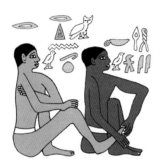

Egyptian foot therapy
A tomb drawing at Saqquara showing a technique similar to modern reflexology.

Reflexology is a complementary therapy in which pressure is applied to the feet or hands to treat a wide range of ailments and to promote psychological well-being and optimum health. The feet and hands are regarded as mirrors of the body, and pressure on specific points (reflexes) found on them treats corresponding areas of the body. Reflexology is holistic and treats each patient as an individual rather than a set of physical symptoms.

History

Forms of foot massage were used by healers in many ancient societies, from Japan to Egypt. Some Native Americans have been using similar methods for centuries. In the early 20th century Dr. William Fitzgerald, an ear, nose, and throat specialist at a US hospital, developed a method of "zone therapy," derived in part from principles outlined in European and other writings. His techniques were developed by another American, Eunice Ingham, who identified and mapped out the reflex zones and was largely responsible for increasing the popularity of what she referred to as "reflexology." Doreen Bayly, one of Eunice Ingham's students, introduced reflexology to the UK in 1960, from where its use spread to other parts of Europe.

This safe and effective form of therapy has since gained increasingly wide acceptance, and its benefits are acknowledged by many within the world of orthodox medicine as well as by its many appreciative recipients.

Key principles

By applying a controlled amount of pressure to specific points on the feet and hands (reflex areas), the therapist can identify and treat problems in all parts of the body. Each precisely defined reflex area is linked to a particular part of the body through a series of longitudinal and transverse zones. The longitudinal zones run though both the legs and the arms, meaning that there are zone-related areas present in certain parts of the body, linking the shoulder and hip, the upper arm and upper leg, the elbow and knee, the forearm and lower leg, the wrist and ankle, and the hand and foot. These may be used as alternative areas for treatment if the affected part cannot be treated directly, because of an injury, for example.

The pressure used in reflexology is not painful, but the recipient may respond with a range of sensations. The therapist uses this feedback to pinpoint the origin of imbalances that are responsible for symptoms.

PRINCIPLES OF REFLEXOLOGY

Reflexologists use the tips of their fingers and thumbs to apply firm, but not heavy, pressure to the reflex areas on the recipient's feet (or sometimes their hands) to assess the state of health of every part of the body. Reflex areas are linked through a carefully defined series of zones to a specific part of the body. Every organ, gland, and other physiological feature has its counterpart in a reflex point, through which the therapist can discover whether the organ or gland is working as it should and apply appropriate pressure to correct any perceived problem. Treatment of the whole body through the feet is given to correct generalized imbalances as part of a complete reflexology session.

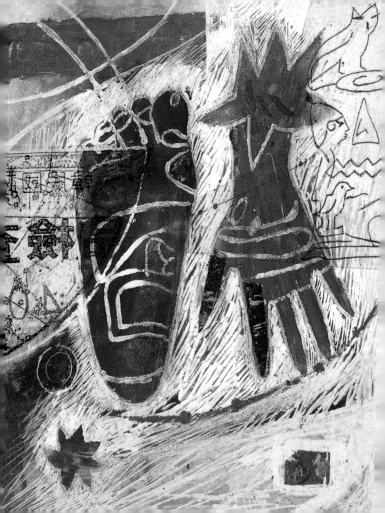

The Evidence for Reflexology

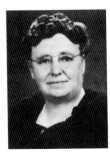

Eunice Ingham
*Ingham was one of the
pioneers of reflexology in
the US in the 1930s.*

Critics of the complementary approach to healing always point out that claims for its effectiveness are not based on the double-blind clinical trials that are used to test new, orthodox forms of treatment. In fact, many medical and surgical treatments have never been subjected to this kind of trial, and doctors have no real understanding of how or why some treatments work. It is also accepted that patients often feel better as a result of the so-called "placebo effect": their symptoms improve because they expect them to, even though the treatment they are being given is actually a "dummy," which has no physiological effect.

Clinical trials

It is impossible to conduct clinical trials on most forms of complementary therapy because of the rules that govern the way such trials are conducted. In a double-blind trial, neither the patient nor the doctor treating him know whether the patient is receiving an active or dummy treatment. Patients are selected for trials on the basis of their conditions and symptoms and compared for other relevant factors, such as smoking or diet. Each is then given an identical form of treatment (or a placebo) and his response compared with that of other people receiving different treatment.

This approach does not lend itself to testing complementary therapies. For one thing, it would be impossible to give reflexology in such a way that neither the therapist nor the recipient knew whether it was the "real thing," nor to give the equivalent of a dummy treatment. Furthermore, reflexology, like most other complementary treatments, is tailored to the whole individual and is thus not the same for everyone, even though they may apparently be suffering from very similar problems.

Response to treatment

The evidence for the effectiveness of reflexology must be of a different kind, and will often depend on observing the response of individuals to treatment. Analysis of replies to a questionnaire sent to its members by the British Reflexology Association (BRA) found that three quarters of them believed their clients improved or recovered from symptoms after treatment. Stress, backache, and sciatica were the most common complaints among the predominantly female clientele. The BRA report suggests that further studies are needed to explore these findings, by defining presenting conditions precisely and measuring the results of treatment.

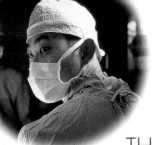

Hospital treatment
Reflexology treatment is now being offered in some health centers alongside conventional treatment.

THE ORTHODOX VIEW

The traditional hostility of orthodox health professionals is no longer as monolithic and unyielding as it once was. An increasing number of doctors and, particularly, nurses, are more open-minded. At the very least, they will concede that it can do no harm, provided the person concerned does not abandon his conventional treatment, and that it may have psychological benefits. At the other end of the spectrum, a growing minority of medically qualified people encourage patients who wish to have reflexology treatment and may arrange for it to be offered in hospital wards or health centers.

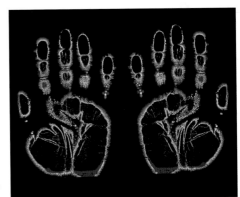

Kirlian photography
This special technique highlights energy changes within the reflex zones.

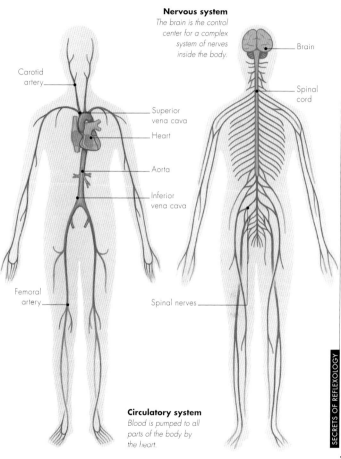

Nervous system

The brain is the control center for a complex system of nerves inside the body.

Brain

Spinal cord

Carotid artery

Superior vena cava

Heart

Aorta

Inferior vena cava

Femoral artery

Spinal nerves

Circulatory system

Blood is pumped to all parts of the body by the heart.

Reflexology and Longitudinal Zones

Dr. William Fitzgerald, one of the pioneers of modern reflexology, identified ten "energy zones," which run vertically through the body from the toes up to the top of the head. There are five such zones on either side of the spine, with end points in each foot and each hand. Zone 1 runs from the big toe, up the inside of the body, and from the thumb along the inside of the arm, to the head. Zone 2 begins at the second toe and the index finger, and the other three zones follow the same pattern, working across the toes and fingers to the outer side of the body. In this way, the body is divided into ten vertical "slices," each of which widens and narrows to an equal degree as it follows the body's contours.

Energy flow

Reflexologists use these zones to gain access to the "energy flow" they believe courses through each, passing through all the parts of the body which lie within

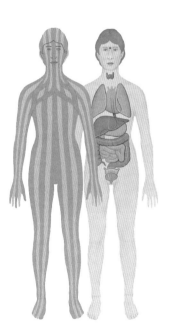

Longitudinal zones
Every part of the body is related to one or more of the energy zones.

each one. If the energy flow becomes blocked or out of balance in any one of these zones, it is thought to affect in turn any part of the body contained within it.

Reflexologists work on different points along the line of the various zones in the feet and hands in order to treat conditions or symptoms resulting from a problem lying along that zone. For example, a reflexologist will work on reflex areas in zone 1 to treat problems that are affecting the spine, neck, nose, and throat.

Meridians

Some practitioners have associated these ten longitudinal zones with the twelve regular meridians, or channels, on which traditional Eastern therapies such as acupuncture and shiatsu are based. However, Eastern therapists work on designated points along the length of all the meridians and not just on the hands and feet.

LONGITUDINAL ZONE MAPS

The zones are usually seen as running from the feet up to the head and down to the hands. Each zone runs through a segment of the body from front to back, and widens and narrows with the body's shape. A reflexology session normally includes treatment of the whole body through the feet and hands, but special efforts can be concentrated in the reflex areas on the hand or foot along the line of the zone where the symptom originates.

Hands and feet

The ten longitudinal zones are represented on the hands and feet, with five zones appearing on the right and five on the left.

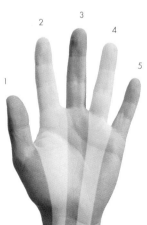

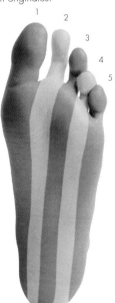

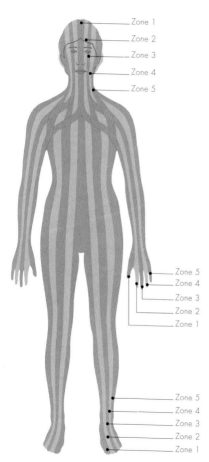

Zone 1
Zone 2
Zone 3
Zone 4
Zone 5

Zone 5
Zone 4
Zone 3
Zone 2
Zone 1

Zone 5
Zone 4
Zone 3
Zone 2
Zone 1

Longitudinal zones

These zones run through
the entire body, from the toes
to the head, and extending
down each arm to the
fingertips. There are five
matching zones on either side
of an imaginary line down
the middle of the body.

Transverse Zones in the Hands and Feet

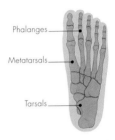

Bones of the feet
The complex structure of the feet makes them extremely versatile.

Phalanges

Metatarsals

Tarsals

In order to pinpoint more accurately the precise areas in the feet and hands that may need to be treated during a reflexology session, a system of transverse zones has been identified to supplement the ten longitudinal zones. These transverse zones lie between lines crossing the feet and hands horizontally, and make it easier for the practitioner to relate sections of the body to the appropriate reflex areas (see pages 22–23). The exact location

of these lines on the feet and hands of any one person will vary slightly, reflecting the differing proportions of an individual's body. For example, the waist line will be closer to the heel on a long-waisted person and farther away on someone who is short-waisted.

Hanne Marquardt, a reflexology therapist working in Germany, was the first to define these guidelines, which make it clear how the horizontal sections of the hands and feet relate to different sections of the rest of the body. Two of the three lines that divide the feet into distinct transverse zones follow the meeting points between specific bands of bones, the third is a notional line between the ankle bones.

Foot zones

The first line is known as the shoulder girdle and follows the junction between the phalanges—the bones of the toes —and the metatarsal bones, which begin at the base of the toes. The second line is the waist line, about halfway along the length of the foot at the point where the metatarsal and tarsal bones meet. The third line, known as the pelvic floor line, crosses the heel between the two ankle bones.

Hand zones

The skeletal structure of the hands does not lend itself quite so readily to easily identifiable transverse zones, although some reflexologists do make use of hypothetical lines visualized on the hands in corresponding positions to those that are mapped on the feet. The area contained within each transverse zone on the hands will be smaller because of the relative size of the hands and feet.

Variations

The locations of the transverse zones vary according to the individual's proportions. In a long-waisted person the waist line is closer to the heel; in a short-waisted person farther away.

TRANSVERSE ZONE MAPS

When you see an illustration of the feet divided up into longitudinal and horizontal zones, the way in which the shape and structure of the foot mirrors that of the rest of the body is more apparent. There is also a degree of symmetry between the overall shape and size of a foot and its owner's body; for example, very tall people are likely to have longer than average feet.

The hands
Some reflexologists visualize "notional" lines on the hands.

The feet
Three lines divide the foot into distinct zones.

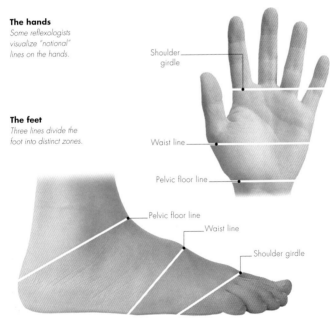

Shoulder girdle

Waist line

Pelvic floor line

Pelvic floor line

Waist line

Shoulder girdle

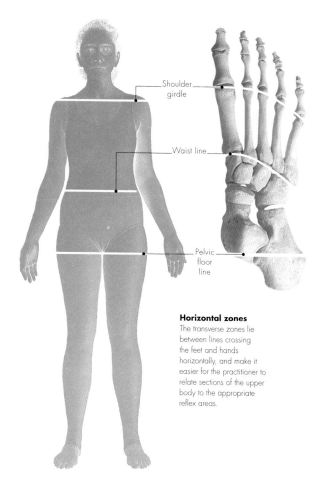

Shoulder girdle

Waist line

Pelvic floor line

Horizontal zones

The transverse zones lie between lines crossing the feet and hands horizontally, and make it easier for the practitioner to relate sections of the upper body to the appropriate reflex areas.

The Effects of an Energy Block

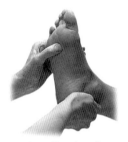

Crystalline deposits
The reflexologist will treat imbalances indicated by "grittiness."

Reflexology treatment is based on the idea that the body has a natural form of energy that, when it flows easily and freely through the zones, helps to maintain optimum health and promote healing. In a healthy person, this energy is dynamic, and balances itself to meet the individual's needs at any given moment. Unfortunately, this ideal state of balanced, free-flowing energy can be easily disrupted, giving rise to all manner of symptoms and conditions or to a generalized lack of well-being. Factors that can have a negative effect on the flow of energy include many aspects of our modern lifestyle.

Orthodox approach

When illness does strike, the first resort is often to the pharmacy or medication prescribed by a doctor. While these treatments may alleviate symptoms, they do not address the problems that caused them in the first place.

Holistic approach

In contrast to this symptom-based approach, a reflexologist will consider the person as an individual and take account of all the factors that may be contributing to their lack of good health when planning treatment. The overall picture will be built up from what the recipient tells him, together with information about specific problem areas sensed through contact with the reflex areas on the feet or hands.

Crystalline deposits

When a particular area is sensitive to pressure or, sometimes, when the therapist can feel a grittiness beneath the skin, as if crystals had been deposited there, this reveals the location of specific imbalances which can then be treated. The more grittiness or tenderness that can be felt, the greater the imbalance.

The reflexologist will try to break down these granular accumulations in order to restore energy flow along the zones and improve blood supply to flush out these "toxins." An experienced reflexologist will be highly sensitive to very subtle imbalances and will plan the treatment that she intends to administer accordingly.

Lifestyle

Many factors, including stress, tension, anxiety, poor diet, environmental pollution, and lack of exercise, can have a negative effect on our natural energy state.

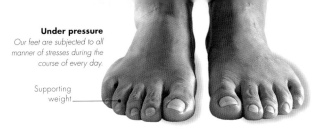

Under pressure
Our feet are subjected to all manner of stresses during the course of every day.

Supporting weight

FUNCTIONS OF HANDS & FEET

Most of us rarely give our hands and feet a second thought unless they begin to trouble us. Healthy feet are strong and flexible, have effective shock absorbers built into the ball of the foot and the heel, and have toes which do a good job of maintaining balance in a variety of situations. The human hand readily adapts to a huge range of tasks, including carrying heavy objects, and making subtle, dexterous, and precise movements.

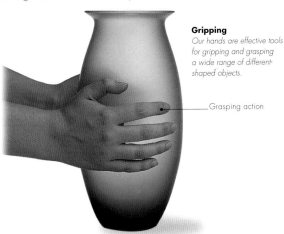

Gripping
Our hands are effective tools for gripping and grasping a wide range of different-shaped objects.

Grasping action

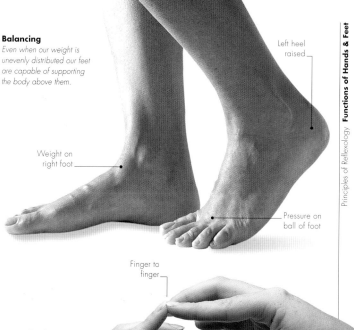

Balancing
Even when our weight is unevenly distributed our feet are capable of supporting the body above them.

Left heel raised

Weight on right foot

Pressure on ball of foot

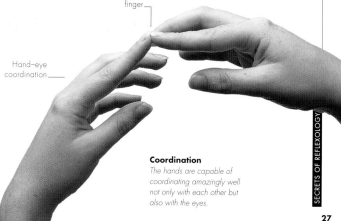

Finger to finger

Hand–eye coordination

Coordination
The hands are capable of coordinating amazingly well not only with each other but also with the eyes.

Foot and Hand Anatomy

The hand and foot have a similar skeletal structure, with 26 bones in the feet and 27 in the hand. When added together, the bones of the feet and hands account for half the total number of bones in our bodies. In the course of our evolution from apes to humans, the functions of the feet and hands have become differentiated, so that we cannot easily walk on our hands nor lift heavy objects with our feet.

Feet

The toes of each foot consist of 14 bones called the phalanges—two in the big toe and three in each of the others. These are attached by ligaments to the long bones, which extend through the foot towards the heel—the metatarsals. The other seven bones are known collectively as the tarsals. Support and stability are provided by three cuneiform bones of the middle of the foot, which

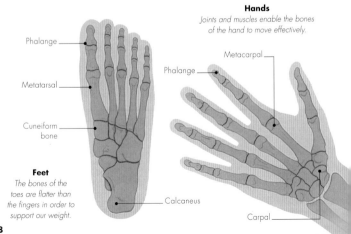

Hands
Joints and muscles enable the bones of the hand to move effectively.

Phalange

Metatarsal

Cuneiform bone

Metacarpal

Phalange

Feet
The bones of the toes are flatter than the fingers in order to support our weight.

Calcaneus

Carpal

connect with the navicular and cuboid bones just in front of the heel. The heel bone is called the calcaneus and the structure is completed by the outer ankle bone—the talus.

This basic structure is given both strength and mobility by a web of 60 to 70 ligaments supporting the joints and about 40 muscles. Potentially vulnerable areas—such as the ball of the foot—are protected and cushioned by layers of fat from the impact of the foot against the ground as we walk, run, and jump.

Hands

The skeletal structure of the hand is very similar to that of the foot. Each hand consists of 27 bones, 14 of which are located in the fingers, five in the palm, and eight in the wrist. Separate joints link each one, enabling the various parts of the hand to perform an astonishingly wide range of complex and delicate movements.

FOOT MAPS
The densest concentration of reflex areas is found on the soles. Parts of the body that are duplicated—such as the kidneys, the lungs, the eyes, and the ears, plus those that are "centered," such as the brain, neck, and stomach—are represented in reflex areas on both feet. Single organs, such as the heart and liver, are only represented on one foot.

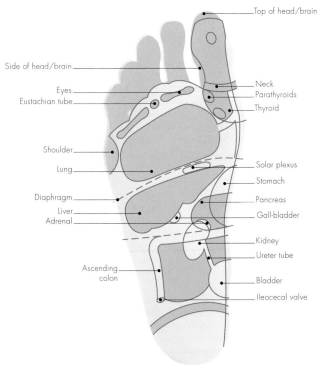

Top of head/brain

Side of head/brain

Eyes
Eustachian tube

Neck
Parathyroids
Thyroid

Shoulder

Lung

Solar plexus
Stomach

Diaphragm
Liver
Adrenal

Pancreas
Gall-bladder

Kidney
Ureter tube

Ascending
colon

Bladder
Ileocecal valve

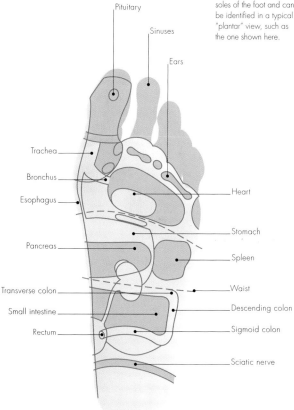

Pituitary

Sinuses

Ears

Trachea

Bronchus

Esophagus

Pancreas

Transverse colon

Small intestine

Rectum

Heart

Stomach

Spleen

Waist

Descending colon

Sigmoid colon

Sciatic nerve

Reflex Points on the Feet

A reflexologist's map of the reflex zones of the feet will show four views—the sole (plantar view), the top (dorsal view), the inside (medial view), and the outside (lateral view). Because the shape of the foot mirrors that of the upper body, the reflex areas are located in corresponding regions:

in other words, the head reflex area is found on the big toe, and the coccyx (tail bone) toward the back of the heel.

All of the reflex areas are very precisely defined, and some are relatively small, so the therapist will need to work like a miniaturist painter when applying pressure to treat them.

DORSAL VIEW

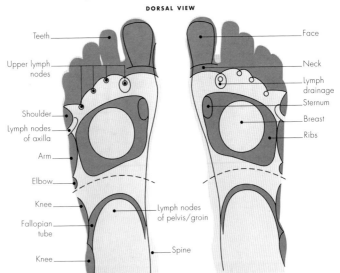

Teeth

Upper lymph nodes

Shoulder

Lymph nodes of axilla

Arm

Elbow

Knee

Fallopian tube

Knee

Face

Neck

Lymph drainage

Sternum

Breast

Ribs

Lymph nodes of pelvis/groin

Spine

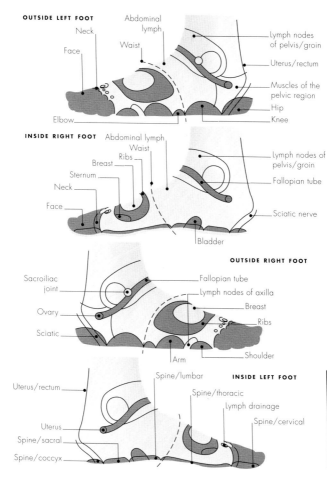

OUTSIDE LEFT FOOT

Neck

Abdominal lymph

Waist

Face

Lymph nodes of pelvis/groin

Uterus/rectum

Muscles of the pelvic region

Hip

Elbow

Knee

INSIDE RIGHT FOOT

Abdominal lymph

Waist

Ribs

Breast

Sternum

Neck

Face

Lymph nodes of pelvis/groin

Fallopian tube

Sciatic nerve

Bladder

OUTSIDE RIGHT FOOT

Sacroiliac joint

Fallopian tube

Lymph nodes of axilla

Breast

Ribs

Ovary

Sciatic

Shoulder

Arm

INSIDE LEFT FOOT

Spine/lumbar

Spine/thoracic

Lymph drainage

Spine/cervical

Uterus/rectum

Uterus

Spine/sacral

Spine/coccyx

HAND MAPS

The reflex areas on the hands mirror those on the feet, although because they have less depth, there is no need for separate maps of the sides of the hands. All the areas can be located on maps of the palm (plantar view) and the back of the hand (dorsal view). The majority of reflex areas are on the palms, and most appear on both hands.

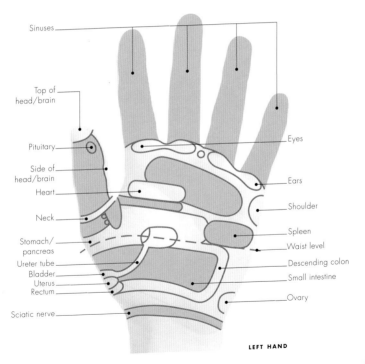

Sinuses

Top of head/brain

Pituitary

Side of head/brain

Heart

Neck

Stomach/pancreas

Ureter tube

Bladder

Uterus

Rectum

Sciatic nerve

Eyes

Ears

Shoulder

Spleen

Waist level

Descending colon

Small intestine

Ovary

LEFT HAND

34

Plantar view

The various parts of the body have their
reflex areas in corresponding regions of the
hands, so, as on the feet, the head area
is found on the tips of the fingers and the
reflex areas for the base of the torso toward
the wrist. Most of the reflex areas occur on
the palms of the hands.

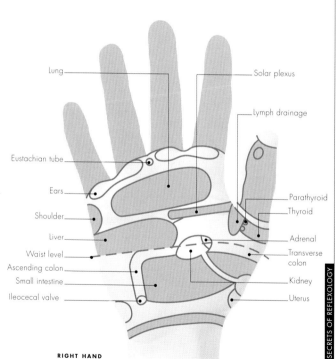

Lung

Solar plexus

Lymph drainage

Eustachian tube

Ears

Shoulder

Liver

Waist level

Ascending colon

Small intestine

Ileocecal valve

Parathyroid

Thyroid

Adrenal

Transverse colon

Kidney

Uterus

RIGHT HAND

Reflex Points on the Backs of the Hands

The reflex areas found on the top of the feet are the same as those on the back of the hand. Some of those shown on the palms extend around the sides of the hand to the backs—such as the diaphragm, hip, and pelvis, and the ovaries and testes, for example.

Although hand treatment is sometimes recommended as a do-it-yourself home treatment, locating the correct areas can be difficult for the inexperienced, because the relative size of the hands compared with the feet means that some areas are in fact very small.

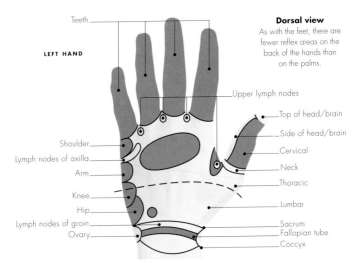

Dorsal view
As with the feet, there are fewer reflex areas on the back of the hands than on the palms.

LEFT HAND

Teeth

Shoulder
Lymph nodes of axilla
Arm
Knee
Hip
Lymph nodes of groin
Ovary

Upper lymph nodes
Top of head/brain
Side of head/brain
Cervical
Neck
Thoracic
Lumbar
Sacrum
Fallopian tube
Coccyx

Sensitivity

The degree to which hands are sensitive to reflexology varies a lot. A reflexologist will sometimes choose to treat the hands in preference to the feet, where there is an injury, deformity, or infection of the feet, for example.

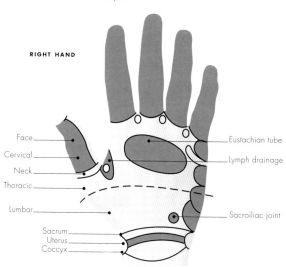

RIGHT HAND

Face
Cervical
Neck
Thoracic
Lumbar
Sacrum
Uterus
Coccyx

Eustachian tube
Lymph drainage
Sacroiliac joint

REFLEXOLOGY BASICS

A reflexology session will generally last between 45 minutes and an hour, although it is likely to be a little shorter if the therapist is working on the hands rather than the feet, the hands being smaller. 🕸️ The reflexologist will generally begin by working the right foot (or hand) first, before turning to the left. This is the sequence recommended by Doreen Bayly. 🕸️ The sensations experienced during treatment vary with the individual, and the degree of pressure applied by the therapist will be adjusted so as to avoid causing pain. She will also take care not to overwork any one area.

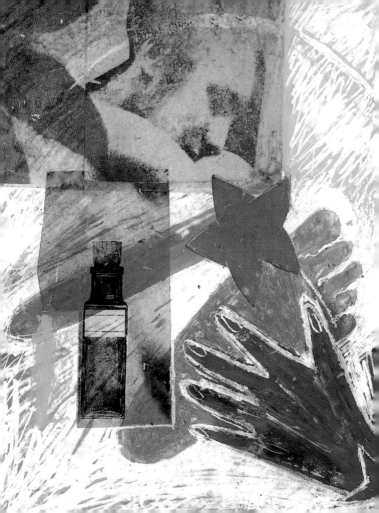

Before a Reflexology Session Begins

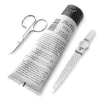

Nail care
The reflexologist must keep her nails trimmed and her hands soft.

Reflexologists always aim to work in parallel with orthodox practitioners when appropriate, so that the patient benefits simultaneously from orthodox and complementary therapy. Before treatment, a reflexologist will question you about your health and lifestyle. There are a few conditions that make reflexology treatment inadvisable—such as deep-vein thrombosis or severe osteoporosis of the feet—and special care is needed in certain instances, for example, when treating people with diabetes, thyroid disorders, pregnant women, or any long-term health problem (see pages 60–61). Tell your reflexologist if you are taking any form of medication (including herbal remedies) since reflexology may interfere with its action.

Preparation

If treating the feet, the reflexologist will ask you to remove your footwear and relax on a couch or in a reclining chair. The reflexologist may use moist wipes to cool and cleanse the feet of any sweat or superficial dirt. She will examine your feet for indications of health problems and will dust them with talcum powder. Then she will give an initial massage to discover areas of tenderness or pain that can be worked on.

Foot problems

The effectiveness of treatment may be diminished if the person's feet are in poor condition. Problems such as corns and calluses should be treated by a podiatrist before going for reflexology.

Blisters and any cuts or abrasions should also be allowed to heal before treatment begins and feet should be moisturized if the skin has a tendency to dryness. If foot problems such as an infection make it either difficult or impossible to treat the feet, then the reflexologist will treat the hands instead, in which case the same principles apply.

Hand care

The therapist's hands are an important "tool of the trade," so like a pianist or a surgeon, she needs to take good care of them. Because she uses the ends of her thumbs (and sometimes fingers) to apply pressure, it is essential that nails are neatly trimmed to avoid digging into the recipient's skin during treatment. The reflexologist will need to keep her hands well moisturized and make sure no patches of hard or rough skin develop, and her hands must always be scrupulously clean.

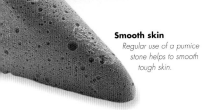

Smooth skin

Regular use of a pumice stone helps to smooth tough skin.

FOOT CARE ROUTINE

After you have washed your feet, take care to dry them thoroughly, especially between the toes. Moisture can encourage fungal infections, such as athlete's foot, to develop. Unless your skin is already very smooth, use a pumice stone and a mildly abrasive cream. Keep your toenails short, and cut them straight across rather than in a curved shape to discourage any tendency to in-grow. Complete your pedicure with plenty of moisturizer.

Nail scissors

Straight cut

Trim toenails

Cutting the nails regularly is important in achieving good foot health.

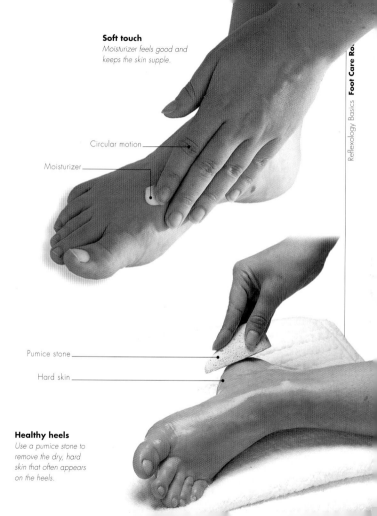

Soft touch
Moisturizer feels good and keeps the skin supple.

Circular motion

Moisturizer

Pumice stone

Hard skin

Healthy heels
Use a pumice stone to remove the dry, hard skin that often appears on the heels.

The Giver–Receiver Relationship

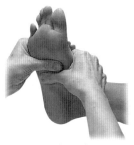

Gentle touch
Many people are nervous at first about being touched.

In any form of therapy, whether orthodox or complementary, treatment is generally more effective if the giver and receiver can establish a good rapport and a trusting relationship. A doctor with a good "bedside manner" can often achieve more than one who is brusque or abrupt; the same applies to any complementary therapist. This means gaining the trust of the receiver and making them feel comfortable so that they are able to relax.

Personal treatment

One of the most important aspects of all kinds of complementary therapy is that it is holistic. Treatment aims to stimulate the body's own self-healing powers and reestablish the body's natural state of balance (homeostasis). Many people say that one of the main reasons why they benefit from reflexology treatment sessions is that they feel they are invited to explain how they really feel, before, during, and after treatment, and that what they say is taken seriously.

Establishing trust

Although reflexology works only on the feet and so does not require undressing completely, just as with massage, many people are still nervous about being touched by a stranger. It helps if the therapist is herself relaxed and calm, and she may need to make a special effort to rid her mind of distracting thoughts so she can focus completely on the person who is consulting her.

Right atmosphere

Many reflexologists are naturally warm
and sympathetic people and good at
listening and putting others at their
ease. Even the most nervous patient
will usually be able to relax once they
realize they are in a safe, nurturing
environment and that the therapist's only
concern is to help them to feel better.
For the receiver, it is important to
understand that reflexology treatment
is a kind of partnership in which both
giver and receiver work together to
help the body and mind regain their
equilibrium to heal themselves.
Treatment is not intended to be a
"magic bullet." Instead, it frees the body
to make use of its own healing and
restorative powers.

Soothing Sounds

To put their patients at ease, some therapists
play soothing music or natural sounds, such as
birdsong or the sound of waves breaking, as
an aid to relaxation and concentration.

THE RIGHT ENVIRONMENT

The reflexologist needs nothing in the way of special equipment, other than suitable seating. The main priorities are warmth, a relaxing atmosphere, and good lighting to enable the therapist to see what she is doing without strain. She may have normal seating to be used in the initial consultation, plus a reclining chair to support the receiver in a comfortable position with her feet raised to a convenient working height.

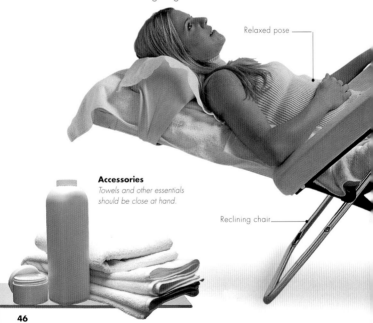

Relaxed pose

Accessories
Towels and other essentials should be close at hand.

Reclining chair

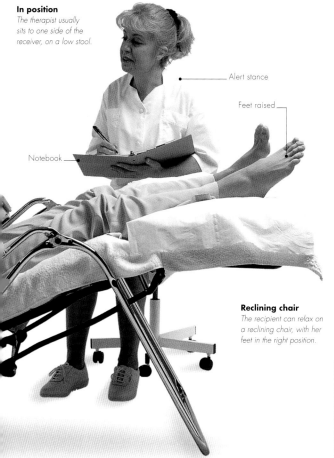

In position
*The therapist usually
sits to one side of the
receiver, on a low stool.*

Alert stance

Feet raised

Notebook

Reclining chair
*The recipient can relax on
a reclining chair, with her
feet in the right position.*

Preparing Mentally

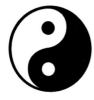

In balance
The therapist must balance her own energy before a treatment.

Once the right environment in which to work has been created, for a reflexologist to make her treatment as effective as it can be, she needs to be calm and relaxed herself before she begins, or she has little chance of inducing her patient to relax. She also needs to be able to concentrate and focus entirely on the work she is doing. Not only does she need to be able to pinpoint reflex areas very precisely, she must also be in the right frame of mind to sense the response of her patient accurately. Because every treatment is tailored to the specific needs of the person concerned, she must be receptive to the nuances of their words

as well as their body language. All this will require a great deal of concentration during treatment.

These requirements place great demands on the therapist and inevitably there will be times when they are not easy to meet. Every individual will have her own methods of clearing intrusive thoughts from her mind and putting aside concerns unrelated to the task before her—yoga and meditation are just two of the established techniques used to promote a calm mind.

Yoga

Many practitioners find techniques drawn from yoga particularly helpful and they can be practiced immediately before a treatment if necessary or whenever it is required. Try adopting the corpse pose, lying flat on your back with your arms away from your sides, palms facing up, and your feet slightly apart. Concentrate on regular breathing, being aware of your abdomen rising and falling as you breathe in and out 20 times or so. Continue breathing slowly and regularly, feeling energy enter your body along with the oxygen.

If you feel tense when you lie down, concentrate on tensing then releasing your muscles, beginning with the toes, and working up the body in stages until you reach your facial muscles.

Meditation

Some people find they can clear their minds by sitting in an empty room and meditating. Various techniques can be used to reach a state of profound relaxation but they all involve the same method: focusing the concentration on a particular activity or image. Each time your mind wanders, consciously bring it back to the point in question; it is difficult to resist intrusive thoughts at first but it gets easier with practice.

Using a Mantra

Some people find it easier to meditate if they have their own mantra, a word or phrase that they repeat continually. The most commonly used mantra is "Om."

THE RIGHT POSITION

The receiver will sit in a comfortable reclining chair that supports the back, neck, and legs. The lower part of the chair is angled so that the knees are slightly bent, with the calves resting comfortably against the support. This places the receiver's feet at a convenient height for the reflexologist to work on them.

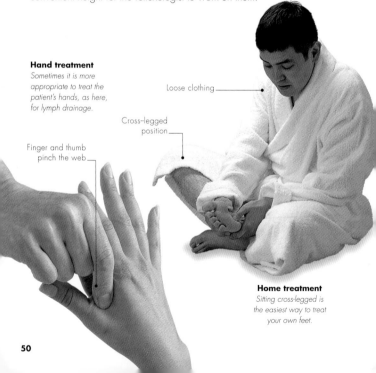

Hand treatment
Sometimes it is more appropriate to treat the patient's hands, as here, for lymph drainage.

Loose clothing

Cross-legged position

Finger and thumb pinch the web

Home treatment
Sitting cross-legged is the easiest way to treat your own feet.

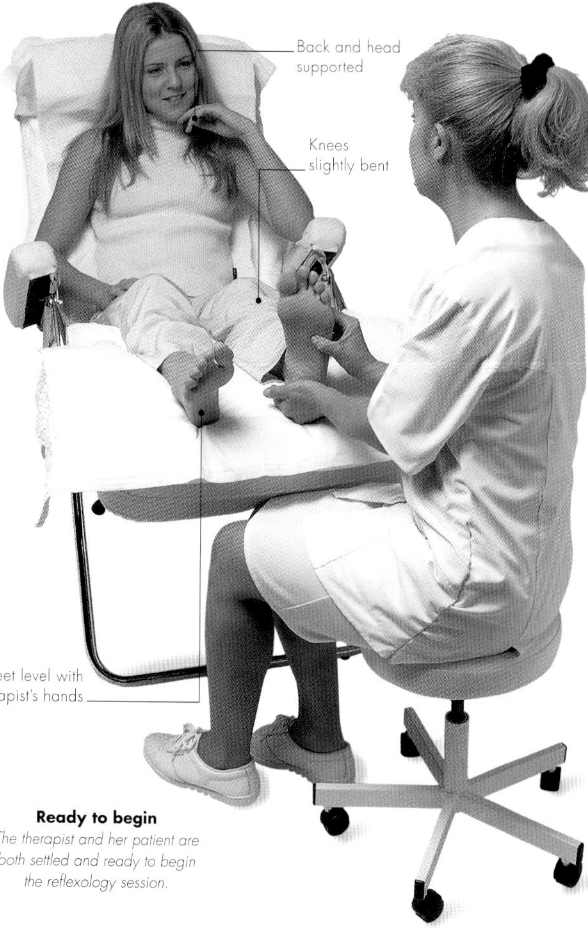

Back and head
supported

Knees
slightly bent

Feet level with
therapist's hands

Ready to begin

*The therapist and her patient are
both settled and ready to begin
the reflexology session.*

Types of Pressure Used in Treatment

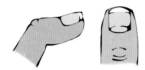

Finger or thumb
Keeping the finger or thumb correctly positioned helps to control the pressure.

Novice reflexologists are often concerned about the amount of pressure to be applied. Too little pressure is likely to be ineffective, while too much may be unpleasant or even, in extreme cases, painful for the receiver. There is no set level of pressure that is appropriate. Instead, it is a matter of the reflexologist adjusting the degree of pressure used according to their observation of the recipient's responses. As a general guideline, the pressure should be firm but not heavy and the therapist should not be conscious of straining in order to press firmly enough.

Individual sensitivity

Individual sensitivity varies widely. Some people will find even relatively light pressure uncomfortable, while others say they can barely feel quite firm pressure. Certain reflex areas are likely to be more tender if the corresponding part of the body is not working properly and so may need a lighter touch.

This issue becomes less significant as the reflexologist gains experience and learns to adjust the level of pressure in response to continuous feedback from the recipient. It may also be necessary to use more pressure when treating the hands as they are often less sensitive than the feet, but some individuals find the opposite is the case.

Thumb movements

During treatment, the thumb (or finger in some instances) should remain in constant touch with the recipient's skin, moving in very small steps from one reflex area to another. Because the distances between points are very small, the movement from one reflex point to another must be very precise. It is important that you avoid straightening the thumb as far as possible. Keeping the thumb bent at the same angle throughout the treatment enables you to apply controlled pressure without strain.

To facilitate this and help the thumb to move smoothly over the skin without dragging, a light coating of talc can be applied to the recipient's foot or hand. In contrast to massage, oil is not applied to the skin in reflexology as this would allow the thumb to slide too easily, making it difficult to apply sustained pressure and to make the tiny movements needed between reflexes.

Technique

A reflexologist's thumb should be kept bent as much as possible, without bending and straightening it again between points.

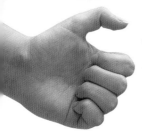

Thumb posture
It is important to avoid straightening the thumb during treatment.

THUMB AND FINGER PRESSURE

Most reflex areas are treated using the thumb, but where this is awkward fingers may be used instead. The position and technique involved are the same. With the thumb bent, pressure is applied with the inner or outer edge rather than the actual tip to avoid the nail pressing into the receiver's skin. Pressure is maintained on the reflex point for a few seconds and then released, and the thumb moves forward to the next point.

Pressure
Pressure is applied to a reflex area using the side of the tip of the thumb, with the thumb bent, held for a few moments, then released.

Movement
Without breaking contact with the recipient's skin, the therapist's thumb moves to the adjacent reflex area in a creeping movement.

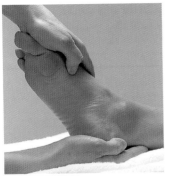

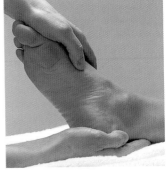

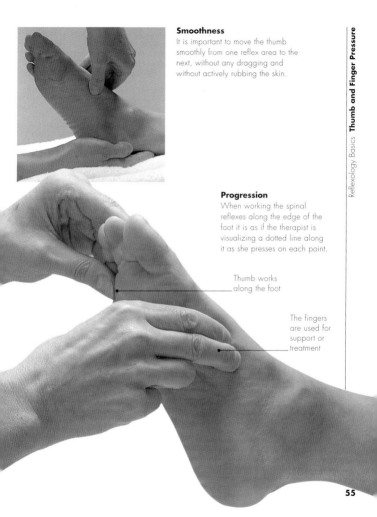

Smoothness

It is important to move the thumb smoothly from one reflex area to the next, without any dragging and without actively rubbing the skin.

Progression

When working the spinal reflexes along the edge of the foot it is as if the therapist is visualizing a dotted line along it as she presses on each point.

Thumb works along the foot

The fingers are used for support or treatment

Maintaining Contact During Treatment

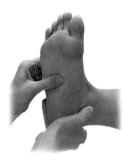

Constant support
The foot must be securely supported with the "non-working" hand.

Reflexologists use a reclining chair for treatment to ensure that the receiver can be comfortable and relaxed, her body well supported, and to place the feet in an easily accessible position. Throughout the session, both the reflexologist's hands should remain in contact with the foot or hand being worked. Any sudden break in contact is disturbing for the receiver and disrupts the seamless flow of the treatment.

Support

As each foot or hand is being worked, it is always supported firmly and comfortably with the therapist's other hand so that the receiver is under no strain and can remain relaxed. As the "working hand" moves around the foot, the position of the supporting hand is adjusted accordingly. The foot can be supported from either side as necessary, and the skin between the thumb and forefinger should be in constant contact with the receiver's foot. The therapist holds the foot so that it is bent slightly toward her, making sure that the toes are never allowed to bend backward. This supporting hand resists the pressure being applied by the working hand, bracing the foot so that it does not move in response to the pressure.

The same principles apply when working the hand, but it is usually easier to support it from below so that it rests comfortably in the palm of the therapist's supporting hand.

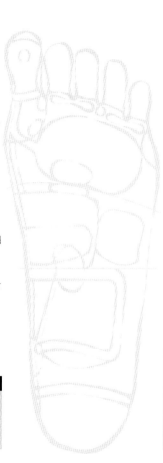

Self-treatment

For self-treatment, the foot can be supported with the free hand, but if you choose to treat your hands rather than your feet, you will need to support the hand on a cushion on your lap.

Right technique

Whether treating yourself or someone else, you must support the foot or hand being worked so that it feels secure and comfortable for the receiver, and so as to allow you to work freely and without any unnatural strain. It may take time for the novice reflexologist to develop the correct technique, but with experience you will begin to sense what feels right for both yourself and the person to whom you are giving treatment.

Reclining Chair

A reclining chair supports the receiver's legs in a relaxed position with the feet raised to a comfortable working height. The therapist may bring a chair if working in the patient's home.

SUPPORTING POSITIONS

The foot must not be allowed to move around and the supporting hand is positioned so as to counter the pressure being applied by the working hand. The foot needs to be held in different positions depending on the reflex being worked, but the basic "hold" is always roughly the same, with the foot resting in the "web" between the forefinger and thumb, and the foot bent slightly toward the therapist.

Neck
This reflex on the sole of the foot (just above where the big toe joins the foot) is worked on the right foot with the right thumb moving from the inside edge, while the left hand supports it.

Transverse colon
This reflex is found on the sole, across all zones at waist level. On the left foot it is worked with the left thumb, with the fingers of the left hand resting on top of the foot.

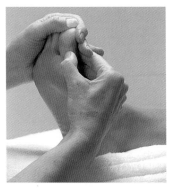

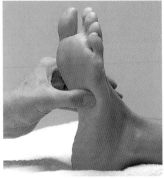

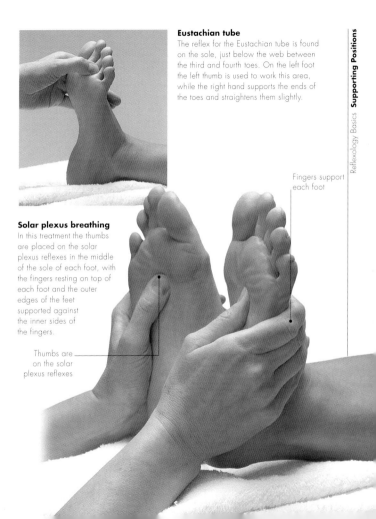

Eustachian tube

The reflex for the Eustachian tube is found on the sole, just below the web between the third and fourth toes. On the left foot the left thumb is used to work this area, while the right hand supports the ends of the toes and straightens them slightly.

Fingers support each foot

Solar plexus breathing

In this treatment the thumbs are placed on the solar plexus reflexes in the middle of the sole of each foot, with the fingers resting on top of each foot and the outer edges of the feet supported against the inner sides of the fingers.

Thumbs are on the solar plexus reflexes

Special Cautions: When Reflexology is Not Suitable

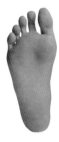

Use with care
Some conditions should not be combined with reflexology.

Reflexology is a true complementary therapy in that therapists often treat those who are receiving orthodox treatment at the same time. They do not claim that reflexology is an alternative to conventional medicine, and would never encourage patients to stop any treatment without consulting their doctor.

However, there are a few conditions in which reflexology is not generally recommended, and others for which treatment should be sought only from an experienced practitioner who is aware of her patient's condition. For example, a reflexologist will postpone giving treatment to someone with a high temperature, a deep-vein thrombosis or phlebitis, or who has just had an operation to replace a joint, until they have recovered. If you are in any doubt about your suitability for treatment, consult your doctor.

Medication
Reflexology is thought to speed up the rate and output of the body's excretions and for this reason may interfere with the action of prescribed medicines. It is essential that the therapist is aware of the fact that treatment can affect the patient's response to medication, such as those used to treat thyroid disorders, diabetes, epilepsy, or hypertension (high blood pressure). Doses may need to be adjusted during a course of reflexology and this is something that the patient must discuss with her medical practitioner. Remember that

reflexology may also interfere with the action of herbal, homeopathic, or aromatherapy treatments.

Pregnancy

Reflexology is not suitable for a woman whose pregnancy is high-risk—if she has had a threatened miscarriage, for example. It is not usually recommended during the first trimester.

Bones and joints

Reflexology is not appropriate for those severely affected by the bone-thinning condition osteoporosis. Conditions such as arthritis and gout that affect the joints (particularly in the hands and feet) may require special precautions, especially if there is inflammation, swelling, or pain.

Self-help in Special Cases

Anyone who is or has been affected by any of the conditions described above should not try to treat themselves; consult a qualified and experienced therapist.

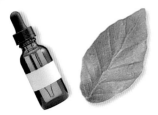

Flower remedies
Bach Flower Remedies can be used to help ease emotional problems.

HELPING YOURSELF
Reflexology does not aim to "cure" illness, but works to enable the body and mind to recover a balanced energy flow and to encourage our own natural healing processes. However, it is asking a lot to expect your body to heal itself if you are do not play your part by looking after yourself. For good health, your body needs the right kind of food and exercise and minimal exposure to environmental pollutants.

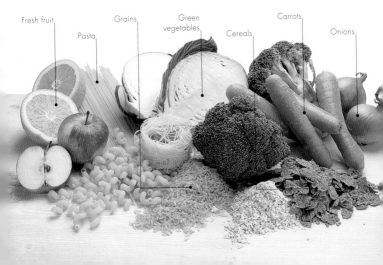

Fresh fruit

Pasta

Grains

Green vegetables

Cereals

Carrots

Onions

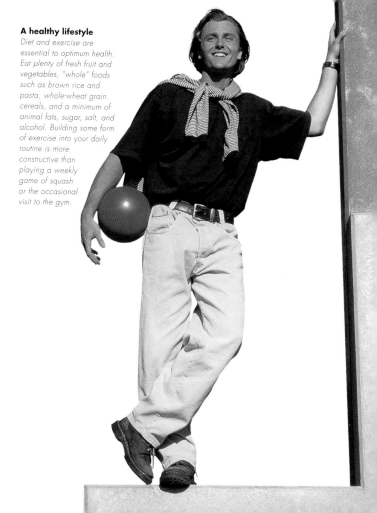

A healthy lifestyle
Diet and exercise are essential to optimum health. Eat plenty of fresh fruit and vegetables, "whole" foods such as brown rice and pasta, whole-wheat grain cereals, and a minimum of animal fats, sugar, salt, and alcohol. Building some form of exercise into your daily routine is more constructive than playing a weekly game of squash or the occasional visit to the gym.

Reflexology and Other Complementary Therapies

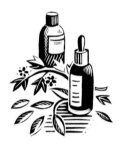

Massage therapy
*Aromatherapy with essential oils
can complement reflexology.*

Reflexology is often used in conjunction with aromatherapy, and, operating on the principle that "more is better," many people decide to try other complementary therapies at the same time as following a course of reflexology treatment. Although the other therapies may indeed have much to offer by way of health benefits, it makes more sense to try them one at a time rather than simultaneously. For one thing, the fact that these therapies may be operating in different ways could

interfere with the effectiveness of each approach but, what is more important, if you do begin to feel better it is difficult to know which one is responsible. However, the benefits of some activities, loosely defined as complementary, may enhance rather than conflict with those of reflexology. These include various movement, touch, and medicinal therapies.

Movement therapies

Yoga, t'ai chi, and the Alexander Technique can all reduce anxiety and muscular tension and aid relaxation, as well as helping to correct postural faults. At least initially, it is better to learn from a qualified and experienced teacher to ensure that you are doing the movements or postures correctly.

Touch therapies

If you have enjoyed the physical contact element of reflexology, you might like to try one of the various forms of massage therapy, such as Swedish massage, Rolfing, or aromatherapy (massage with essential oils). These therapies boost the circulatory and immune systems and can enhance your overall feeling of well-being dramatically. Touch therapies can be beneficial for chronic problems such as backaches and insomnia.

Medicinal therapies

If you feel your problems have an emotional basis, Bach Flower Remedies may be a good choice, and you can use them to treat yourself. Physical and psychological symptoms often respond well to treatment from a homeopath, and although it is possible to treat yourself safely, the results may not be as good. The range of herbal remedies now available for self-treatment is enormous, but because some of them have powerful effects and the strength and purity of different brands vary, it is wise to have an initial consultation with an herbalist if possible.

A BASIC FOOT
REFLEXOLOGY SESSION

During a treatment session, the reflexologist will work on all the reflex points on both feet, usually starting with the right foot. As she does so, she will spend additional time on any areas relating to specific symptoms or those where tenderness indicates that the particular part of the body is not working as it should. She will be guided in this by the responses of the person she is treating as each area is worked in turn. ✍ At the end of the session, she may return to work any problem areas again, before finishing with foot relaxation and solar plexus breathing sequences.

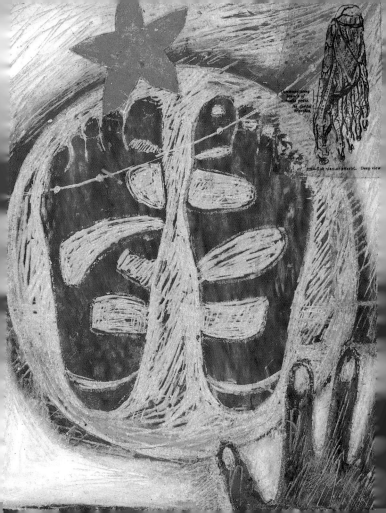

Full Foot Workout

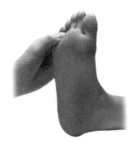

Top down
Treatment moves from the top of the foot down to the ankle.

During a treatment session of around an hour, all the reflex areas on both feet will be worked thoroughly, with the therapist spending more time on any areas which are important for the individual being treated. She will concentrate on these areas as she comes to them, and may work them again toward the end of the session. If they felt tender when first treated, this may be less noticeable when they are worked again if the related part of the body has begun to respond to treatment.

Order of treatment

Practitioners vary in the order in which they choose to treat; some beginning with the right foot and some with the left; some work alternately on each foot, working a few areas at a time. Although the different approaches all have their own rationale, many therapists follow the order introduced by the pioneers of reflexology, Eunice Ingham and Doreen Bayly, and complete the treatment of the right foot before working on the left.

The advantages of this approach include the fact that the first parts of the large intestine, which are represented on the right foot, are treated before the final parts on the left foot. It also means that treatment of the heart, which is represented only on the left foot, is not begun until well into the session, when the individual has had time to get used to the treatment and relax.

Reflexology treatment begins at the top of the body, that is to say, the head and brain. These parts of the body are represented in the big toes. Treatment

then moves down through the other
areas, working each area in order from
the toes toward the ankles.

Differences between feet

While many parts of the body are
represented in both feet, certain organs
only appear on one, which means there
is some difference in the way each foot
is worked. Important parts of the body
that are not represented on both feet
include the liver, gallbladder, and the
ascending colon (all on the right foot
only), and the heart, spleen, rectum,
and the transverse, descending, and
sigmoid colon (on the left foot only).
Thus if an individual has problems that
indicate a blockage in a part of the
body related to a specific area on one
foot, such as the spleen, this may be
treated several times in one session.

Whole Body

Wherever the particular therapist chooses to
begin a treatment, the most important rule is
that every part of the body should be worked
on the feet.

RIGHT FOOT 1 • PRACTICE

Working the head reflexes can help to ease symptoms such as headaches and those arising from conditions with a psychological component, such as insomnia. The pituitary gland plays an important role in controlling and regulating hormone balance. The neck area may be important if the person is experiencing headaches or has any injury or stiffness. Problems in the spine can cause a range of symptoms, including backaches.

Top of head

The reflex area for the top of the head and the top of the brain is located across the fleshy part at the top of the big toe, just behind and below the nail.

Side of head

The reflex area for the side of the head and the side of the brain is located on the side of the big toe, alongside the second toe of the foot.

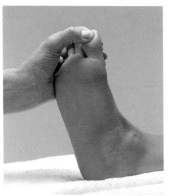

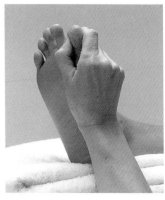

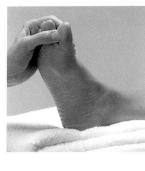

Pituitary gland

On the underside of the big toe is a fleshy pad and in the center of this the reflex for the pituitary gland is located.

Neck

The front and back of the neck are represented on the front and back respectively of the big toe, at the base where the toe meets the foot.

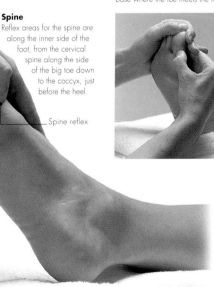

Spine

Reflex areas for the spine are along the inner side of the foot, from the cervical spine along the side of the big toe down to the coccyx, just before the heel.

Spine reflex

Right Foot 2 • Theory

Head treatment
Many conditions benefit from treatment to the head areas.

The reflexologist is likely to spend a considerable amount of time working the various reflexes around the big toe and the point where it joins the sole of the foot because of the relatively large number of reflex areas represented in this area. In addition to the head and the brain, other important organs and structures in or on the head are to be found in this region. These may be significant for a number of reasons, and can be implicated in many conditions and symptoms, both physical and psychological. Many of these reflexes are extremely small and require great precision when working.

Face

The face is well supplied with nerves, which may be responsible for problems such as neuralgia. The teeth and gums reflex areas may need extra treatment for symptoms such as toothaches or a gum infection.

Sinuses

The sinuses in the skull both above the eyes and behind the cheeks may become congested or infected, causing pain and/or breathing difficulties. The reflexes for these parts of the body are around the sides and bases of the toes and may need treatment following a severe cold or if the person suffers from a chronic infection.

Eustachian tube

Any upper respiratory tract infection, phlegm, or an allergic condition such as hay fever or rhinitis, may result in the Eustachian tube (which connects the throat and the ear) becoming blocked. As a result, this can affect a person's ability to hear properly.

Ears and eyes

The ear and eye reflexes are located where the toes meet on the sole of the foot. Any or all of these reflexes may need additional treatment if the person receiving treatment has any kind of problems with her vision or hearing or sometimes, in the case of the ears, with balance or dizziness.

Even when the person being treated does not have symptoms related to or arising from these areas, it is important to devote careful attention to all of them so as to ensure that they are working as well as possible.

Any disruption of or imbalance in the energy flow in these areas can leave a person feeling below par and may reflect an overall level of tension that stops the body from working as well as it should.

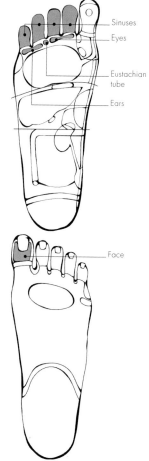

Sinuses

Eyes

Eustachian tube

Ears

Face

Further Information

For further information about treatment for conditions affecting these parts of the body, see pages 156–157, 176–177, and 180–181.

RIGHT FOOT 2 • PRACTICE

Many of these reflexes are relatively small and will need to be worked very precisely, although conditions such as allergy or an infection, which produce varied symptoms in several of these organs and structures, mean they will all need thorough treatment. Treatment for any problems involving the face, including the mouth, lips, eyes, ears, and nose, will involve working this area as well as the specific reflexes for those parts.

Face

The reflex area for the face is found on the front of the foot, below the nail on the big toe. The teeth are represented on the top of the foot, just below the toenails and range through zones 1 to 5, according to their position in the jaw.

Sinuses

The reflexes for the sinuses are represented up the sides and back of the toes. Depending on which ones are affected—those on the cheeks (the maxillary sinuses) or those above the eyes (the frontal sinuses)—treatment will concentrate on the relevant areas.

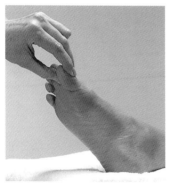

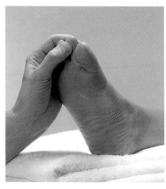

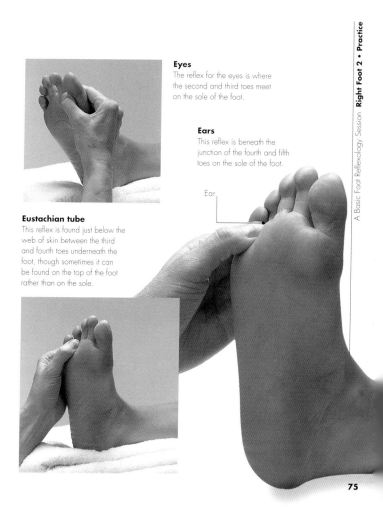

Eyes
The reflex for the eyes is where the second and third toes meet on the sole of the foot.

Ears
This reflex is beneath the junction of the fourth and fifth toes on the sole of the foot.

Ear

Eustachian tube
This reflex is found just below the web of skin between the third and fourth toes underneath the foot, though sometimes it can be found on the top of the foot rather than on the sole.

Right Foot 3 • Theory

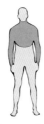

The upper body

Reflex areas for many vital organs as well as the arms and shoulders will be treated.

When working the reflexes for the upper part of the body, the therapist will look for signs of blocked or unbalanced energy flow and slight tenderness in these areas is not uncommon.

Shoulder and arm

When working the shoulder and arm reflexes, it is essential to pay attention to the main joints, including the shoulder, the elbow, and the wrist, to encourage a full range of movement. Tension or injuries affecting the muscles will be felt as tenderness in the relevant reflexes.

Thyroid

The thyroid gland in the front of the neck regulates various aspects of the metabolism. If the thyroid gland is not working properly, the person is likely to feel generally under par.

Lungs

Good lung function is vital because this is the source of the oxygen needed by every cell in the body, and also the means by which waste carbon dioxide is expelled. Any problems affecting the lungs may result in an insufficient supply of oxygen to more distant parts of the body. A number of conditions, such as asthma, bronchitis, and upper respiratory tract infection, can stop the lungs from working to their full capacity, and stress and anxiety can sometimes inhibit normal breathing.

Solar plexus

When treating a person who is affected by stress, the reflexologist will pay special attention to the reflex area for the solar plexus, a network of nerves located in the upper abdomen just below the diaphragm, to encourage thorough relaxation. The solar plexus reflex is important when treating any symptoms related to stress or anxiety, and also in promoting energy balance, and mental and physical relaxation.

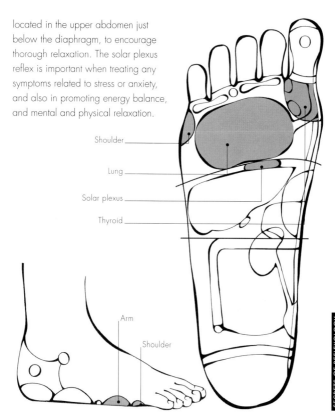

Shoulder

Lung

Solar plexus

Thyroid

Arm

Shoulder

RIGHT FOOT 3 • PRACTICE

Thorough treatment of these reflexes is important as part of a full treatment, and many people experience problems in these areas at some time, whether as a result of injury, illness, or stress. As well as treating the appropriate reflex areas, any problems in this part of the body may also benefit from treatment to the zone-related area—the ankle for the wrist or the knee for the elbow, for example.

Shoulders

The shoulder reflex area is represented on the sole and the top of the foot, around the base of the little toe.

Arms

The reflexes for the arm extend down the outer edge of the top of the foot, with the elbow halfway between the toes and the heel.

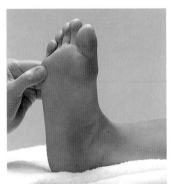

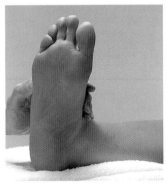

Thyroid

The thyroid gland is represented around the ball of the foot, just below the big toe.

Solar plexus

The reflex for the solar plexus is found on the sole of the foot, just below the diaphragm level in zones 2 and 3.

Solar plexus

Lungs

Adjacent to the thyroid, over the ball of the foot below the second to fifth toes, is a relatively large reflex representing the lungs.

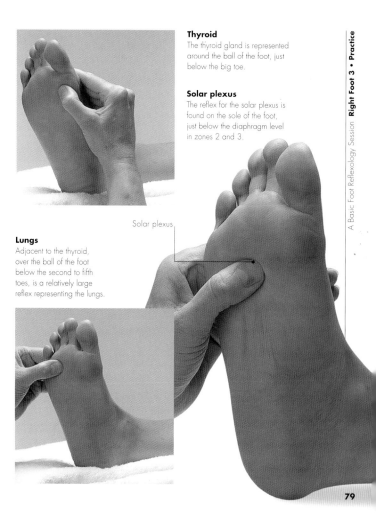

Right Foot 4 • Theory

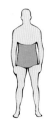

The lower body

These reflexes are especially important for digestive symptoms.

As she works the abdominal area and the lower part of the trunk, the reflexologist will know that many organs within the digestive and immune systems are located in this part of the body. The reflexes for the liver, gallbladder, and part of the large intestine are only found in the right foot, while others, such as those for the kidneys and bladder, are on both feet.

Liver

The liver is the body's largest internal organ, and if it is not working properly, the person may experience a general feeling of malaise or specific symptoms, such as yellowing of the skin and the whites of the eyes, and digestive problems. The liver reflex is very large, crossing all five zones on the sole of the foot. The gallbladder, attached to the right side of the liver, plays an important role in fat digestion and stores the bile produced by the liver.

Stomach

Everything we eat and drink arrives in the stomach where the vital process of digestion begins, but problems in this area are so common as to be almost universal. Nearly everyone experiences stomachaches and indigestion at some point, particularly when they are under stress, eat the wrong kinds of food, or grab snacks "on the run."

Large intestine

The right foot is usually treated before the left because this is where the reflexes for the first part of the large intestine are represented. The therapist can work the various parts of the colon in the order in which the products of digestion travel through it, thus encouraging the natural flow through the body. Any fluid not needed by the body is filtered and then transmitted by the kidneys to the bladder, where it is stored until it can be passed out as urine.

Sciatic nerve

The sciatic nerve begins in the lumbar and sacral spine areas and passes through the buttocks to the thighs, and down to the knees. Problems affecting this nerve can cause excruciating pain.

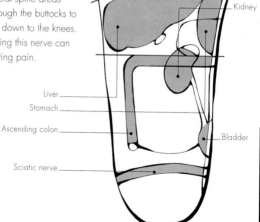

Kidney

Liver

Stomach

Ascending colon

Bladder

Sciatic nerve

RIGHT FOOT 4 • PRACTICE

Thorough treatment of the liver and gallbladder areas encourages the body to make the best use of vital nutrients in the diet, maintaining a good supply of "fuel" for energy and controlling body temperature. The entire large intestine needs to be working well to ensure that the body extracts all the water it needs from the diet and to ensure that waste matter can be excreted efficiently.

Liver

The liver reflex is on the sole of the right foot, between the waist and diaphragm levels, and crosses all five zones, narrowing as it reaches the inner edge of the foot. The gallbladder adjoins the liver in zone 3 of the right foot.

Stomach

The left foot reflex is most important for treating the stomach, but this area of the body may also be represented on the sole of the right foot in zone 1, between the waist and diaphragm levels.

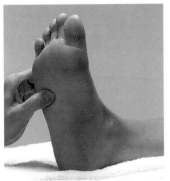
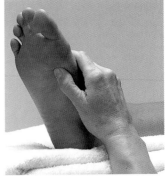

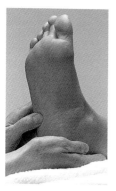

Large intestine

The reflexes for various elements of the large intestine are represented in areas on both feet. The ascending colon and part of the transverse colon are to be found on the right foot.

Kidney

The kidney reflex is on the sole of the foot at the level of the waist line in zones 2 and 3.

Bladder

Working the kidneys and bladder, on the sole and edge of the foot respectively, helps the body to eliminate any unwanted fluid in the form of urine.

Sciatic nerve

Across the pad of the heel is the reflex for the sciatic nerve; there is an additional reflex on either side of the Achilles tendon.

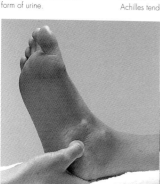

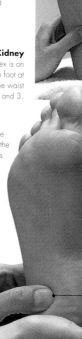

Sciatic nerve

Left Foot Theory

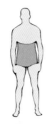

Single organs
Reflexes for the heart and spleen are only found on the left foot.

When the reflexologist moves onto the left foot, she will work all the reflexes that were worked on the right foot, plus those that are only represented on this foot. These include the heart, spleen, and the final parts of the colon.

As before, the reflexologist will begin by working the head and brain and the reflexes represented on or just below the toes, working her way systematically down the left foot (and thus the body), just as she did previously on the right side. Again, she will devote extra time and attention to any reflexes that appear to be especially sensitive, indicating that the related part of the body is not working as well as it should.

She will also take extra care to work those reflexes that are relevant to particular symptoms or signs of energy imbalance, which are being experienced by the patient. Some reflexes on the left foot may need extra attention if there is a problem that relates specifically to that side of the body—such as a knee or hip joint, for example.

Heart

Although the position of the heart within the body is toward the left side (in the vast majority of people), it does extend into zone 1 on the right side. However, it is represented only in the left foot, in zones 2 and 3.

Working the heart reflex can have a beneficial effect on the blood circulation in general. Treatment can also help with specific conditions such as angina. Furthermore, it may help to prevent heart problems from developing in the future in a person who is healthy.

Spleen

Treating the spleen will help to keep the immune system functioning well because this organ plays an important role as the source of lymphocytes, the white blood cells that attack invading infectious organisms. It is located on the left side of the body, just above waist level, and its reflex is found in the left foot.

Large intestine

The reflex areas for the final parts of the large intestine—the extension of the transverse colon, the descending and sigmoid colons, and the rectum—are all only found in the left foot.

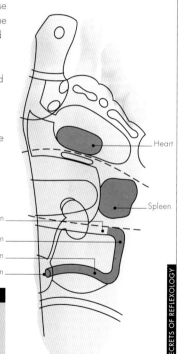

Heart

Spleen

Transverse colon

Descending colon

Sigmoid colon

Rectum

Treating the Heart Reflex

Treatment to the heart reflex should only be given by an experienced reflexologist; it must be done with great care. Extra caution is needed for treating specific heart conditions.

LEFT FOOT • PRACTICE

The reflexes for the various elements that make up the reproductive system are found on both feet, with the same areas representing different male and female organs. Other important points to treat, which are found on top of the foot, represent the lymphatic nodes. Like the spleen, the lymphatics are a vital component of the immune system, and treating the reflexes in both feet is essential if the body is to defend itself effectively against infection.

Heart
Although the heart itself is located partly in the right side of the body, the reflex area for the heart is only found in zones 2 and 3 of the left foot, just above the diaphragm level.

Knee
This important and complex joint is represented on the outer edge of the foot, in a semicircular area beginning around the waist line and extending halfway toward the heel.

Hip
The reflex area for the hip will also be treated for problems arising in the top part of the leg. It is found on the outer edge of the foot, from the heel to the knee reflex in a semicircular shape.

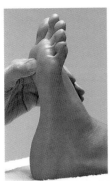
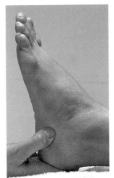
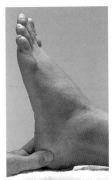

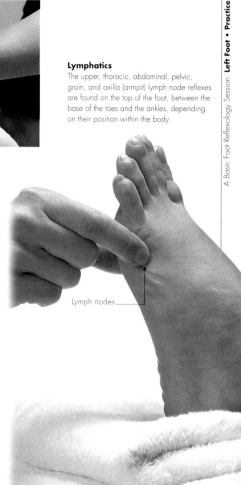

Lymphatics
The upper, thoracic, abdominal, pelvic, groin, and axilla (armpit) lymph node reflexes are found on the top of the foot, between the base of the toes and the ankles, depending on their position within the body.

Lymph nodes

Uterus/prostate
These reflexes are on the other side of the foot, at the same level as the ovary/testis.

Ovary/testis
These are on the outer edge of the foot, midway between the back of the heel and the tip of the ankle bone.

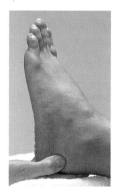

Foot Relaxation

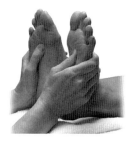

Easing tension

*Foot exercises relax the
receiver after treatment has
been completed.*

By the time each foot has been
thoroughly worked at the end of
a treatment session, they should
both be completely relaxed and flexible
and thus will be able to move very
easily and freely. This is why a series
of general exercises to reinforce the
relaxing effect of treatment are
performed during the final phase of the
session. Although this is an essential
part of a reflexology session, foot
relaxation does not take very long to
do, and will comprise only about three
minutes out of the whole treatment time.

Exercise routine

The exercises reinforce the overall effect
of the treatment and help the receiver
to "come to" once her treatment is
completed. Some reflexologists
may perform these exercises at the
beginning of a session as well,
particularly if the receiver is nervous
about the forthcoming treatment or is
especially tense and anxious. It may
also be helpful to begin with these
exercises if parts of the feet are tender
or hypersensitive because some parts
of the body are not working properly.

As each part of the foot is exercised
in turn, it has a stretching effect on the
related part of the body, helping to
eliminate any remaining tension and
stiffness.

The process (see page 90–91)
begins with the toes, each of which is
rotated, first in one direction, then in the
other. This will relieve any tension in the
neck area. In particular, if the big toe
joint is very stiff, this could indicate that
the recipient's neck is also stiff. It is
important that the toe is not rotated too

quickly, since this could make the patient feel very dizzy: it is the equivalent of rotating the head very fast.

The therapist then works along the length of each foot, first using a wringing action—the equivalent of pulling back the shoulders and spreading out the organs within the chest and abdominal cavity. The next stage is kneading the sole of the foot. Here the therapist is working the diaphragm itself and the whole of the rest of the body. Finally the ankles are very gently rotated, first in one direction and then in the other. It is essential that it is the practitioner and not the patient who controls this rotation to ensure that the ankle remains relaxed. Gentle rotation will help to loosen any stiffness in the pelvic area and stimulate the free flow of energy throughout the body.

Timing

These exercises are best performed at the end of the treatment of each foot, because the foot will then be in a relaxed state and the movements can be performed without strain.

FOOT RELAXATION STEP-BY-STEP

While performing the treatment, the therapist needs to be constantly checking her hold to ensure that the receiver is comfortable and relaxed and that she herself is able to support the foot or hand being worked without any awkwardness or physical strain. It is important to support the foot correctly when the exercises are being performed to promote relaxation and avoid any sense of strain or discomfort for the receiver.

Toe rotation
When the toes are being worked by holding the top of each toe in turn, the other hand holds the base of the toes in a secure grip to support the joints between the metatarsals and the phalanges.

Wringing
Both hands are used for the wringing action. One hand supports the foot from below, with the fingers around the outside and resting on the top, while the other hand is held around the inner edge; both thumbs are on the sole.

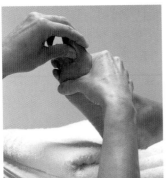

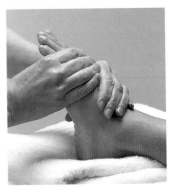

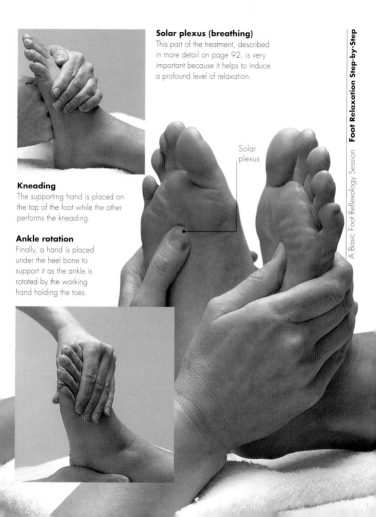

Solar plexus (breathing)
This part of the treatment, described in more detail on page 92, is very important because it helps to induce a profound level of relaxation.

Solar plexus

Kneading
The supporting hand is placed on the top of the foot while the other performs the kneading.

Ankle rotation
Finally, a hand is placed under the heel bone to support it as the ankle is rotated by the working hand holding the toes.

Closing Down after Foot Reflexology

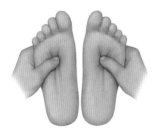

Final phase
Solar plexus treatment brings the session to a conclusion.

To bring the active part of the treatment session to a close, a final exercise called solar plexus breathing is done.

Solar plexus breathing

The therapist holds both feet, with her hands around the outer edges about halfway down each foot. She rests her fingers on the top of each foot, with her thumbs on the solar plexus reflex points on the sole. As the receiver inhales deeply, she applies firm pressure to the two solar plexus reflexes, gently easing the feet upward and toward the receiver at the same time. The receiver then exhales and, as she slowly releases the air, the pressure on the solar plexus reflexes is relaxed and the feet are eased down gently again.

This sequence is then repeated four or five times, to allow the therapist to check the receiver's breathing and encouraging complete relaxation as the treatment finally comes to an end.

Discussion and planning

The last few minutes of the session is then spent in talking over what has been achieved and what should happen next. This is an opportunity to exchange experiences: how the receiver felt while the treatment was taking place, how she feels now, and what the reflexologist has learned about the receiver's health and any energy imbalances. Future treatment sessions can be planned if required, and the therapist will also explain what responses to the treatment may develop over the next few hours or days. It may help the patient to keep a diary to monitor the effects of treatment.

Side effects

Individuals react in different ways, but common minor side effects include slight nausea, a runny nose as the sinuses clear, and the need to empty the bladder or bowels more frequently as toxins are eliminated. Some people feel tired for a day or so after treatment, but others may feel energized. Any such effects normally wear off after 24 to 48 hours and are often a sign that the treatment is having a real effect.

Healing Crisis

A temporary relapse in health, or "healing crisis," often indicated by a cough or rash, is seen as a sign that the body is ridding itself of toxins, but could also indicate overtreatment.

A BASIC HAND
REFLEXOLOGY SESSION

A reflexologist may decide to treat the hands if the feet cannot be treated easily or effectively for some reason: perhaps because of a widespread infection or an injury, or occasionally because the person being treated dislikes having their feet massaged, possibly because they are very sensitive or ticklish. ✍ The session will follow the same course, but will be shorter because of the relatively small size of the hands compared with the feet, and may not be quite as effective. ✍ Many people who like to treat themselves find it easier to work on their hands because they are more accessible.

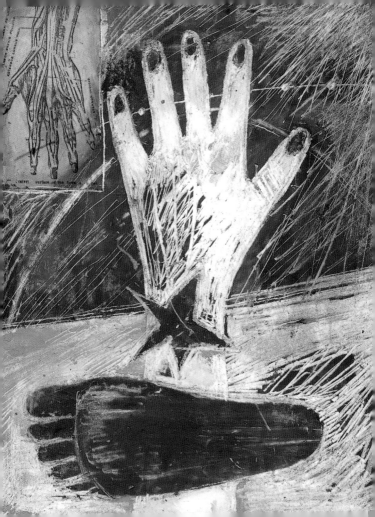

Full Hand Workout

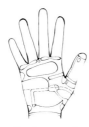

Hand treatment

*A full body treatment on
the hands should ideally
be done by a reflexologist.*

The principles that govern
reflexology treatment to the hands
are the same as those for treating
the feet. The longitudinal zones are
arranged in just the same way, ranging
from zone 1 on the inner side by the
thumb to zone 5 at the outer edge, just
by the little finger. The transverse zones
are less significant in the hands, and do
not have the same clear relationship to
their skeletal structure as the transverse
zones in the feet. Because the hands
are smaller than the feet, it is more
difficult to locate some reflex areas,
especially the smaller ones.

Treatment

During a treatment session, all the reflex
areas on both hands will be worked
thoroughly. If reflex areas felt tender
when they were first treated, this may
be less noticeable when they are
worked again if the related part of
the body has since begun to respond
to treatment.

A reflexology treatment on the hands
takes less time than one on the feet
because there is less surface area to
cover. The fact that hands are smaller
than feet means that the reflex areas
are correspondingly smaller, and the
reflexologist will need to work with even
greater accuracy and precision when
treating the hands.

Self-treatment

Although many reflexes are easier to
reach on the hands for self-treatment,
the difficulty of pinpointing the smaller
areas accurately means that it is really
only practical to give some symptomatic
treatment, and a full body treatment is
best done by a reflexologist. However,

hands are much more convenient for a self-help session and can be practiced at any time, whether as an additional treatment between foot reflexology sessions or to bring temporary relief for conditions such as stress, for example.

Order

Some reflexologists may prefer to begin with the left hand or work alternately on reflexes in each hand, but most will opt to begin with the right hand before moving onto the left, perhaps returning to treat difficult areas again toward the end of the session.

Treatment will first be given to the head and brain, represented on the top and sides of the thumb. The therapist will work her way progressively down the hand, treating points on both sides as she moves toward the wrist.

Differences

While most parts of the body are represented in both hands, some major organs and structures are only found on one hand, such as the heart and the liver.

RIGHT HAND 1 • PRACTICE

Treating the pituitary gland helps to regulate production of all the hormones released by the endocrine glands and adjust the balance between them. The other structures in the head are also treated, including the rest of the brain, followed by the cervical and thoracic spine. These areas are important for any kind of headache, including migraines, for pain and stiffness in the neck itself, and for pain in the middle of the back.

Top of head

The reflex for the top of the head and the area of the brain underlying it is found on the fleshy part of the thumb, just behind and below the thumbnail.

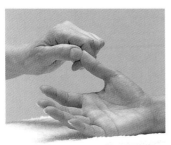

Side of head

The side of the head and the related part of the brain are represented in a reflex area located on the inner side of the thumb, alongside the forefinger.

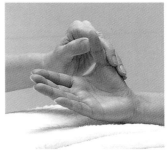

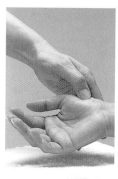

Thoracic spine
The thoracic spine is represented on the inside of the hand, just below the base of the bone in the thumb.

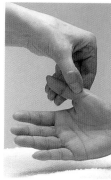

Neck
The front and back of the neck are represented in reflex areas on the front and back respectively at the base of the thumb, where it meets the hand.

Pituitary
The pituitary gland, sometimes described as the "conductor of the hormone orchestra," is represented in the center of the fleshy pad of the thumb.

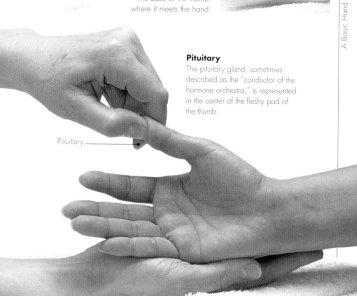

Pituitary —

Right Hand 2 • Theory

The head

All the reflexes in this area must be treated with considerable accuracy.

As she works on the reflexes for the face, the reflexologist will be treating some very small areas, such as those for the Eustachian tube (which links the ear and throat) and the sinuses (the air-filled spaces in the skull, above and below the eyes), and will need to work with great precision.

Face, teeth, and gums

Treating the face area will help to relax tense muscles and alleviate pain such as neuralgia, as well as relieving minor but unpleasant problems such as canker sores and cold sores. Working the reflex areas for the teeth and gums will keep them healthy, and may help in cases of toothaches and gum disease.

Sinuses and Eustachian tube

The sinuses and the Eustachian tube (also known as the auditory tube) need to be clear. They can sometimes become congested or infected following an upper respiratory tract infection such as a cold, or an allergy such as rhinitis, causing pain, breathing problems, and difficulty with hearing.

Eyes and ears

Moving from the thumb down into the palm of the hand, the reflexologist will treat the areas representing the eyes and ears. The aim is to reduce any blockage or imbalance of energy so as to enable the person to see and hear as well as possible and prevent problems from developing.

Reflexology treatment can also help to ease the symptoms of eye irritation, conjunctivitis, or sties. Treating the ear reflex can help the body to fight off an infection, ease earaches and tinnitus (buzzing in the ears), and improve any problems a person may have with balance or dizziness.

When performed in conjunction with treatment to the brain area, treating the eyes or ears may also help a person with limited vision or hearing to interpret what they can see or hear to the full extent of their capabilities.

If there are specific symptoms associated with these parts of the body, the reflexologist may want to treat these reflexes again once she has worked all the other reflexes in the hands.

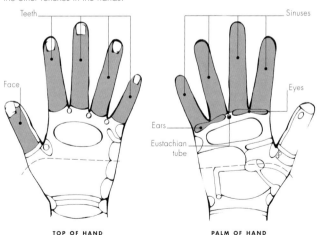

Teeth

Sinuses

Face

Eyes

Ears

Eustachian tube

TOP OF HAND

PALM OF HAND

RIGHT HAND 2 • PRACTICE

The reflex area for the face is just under the base of the thumbnail. In the same position, on the backs of the fingers, are the teeth reflexes. The Eustachian tube is usually just below the point where the third and fourth fingers meet, where the palm begins. Beneath the other fingers are small reflex areas representing the eyes and ears. The sinuses reflex areas are on the front and sides of the fingers.

Face

The reflex area for the face can be found under the base of the thumbnail, on the back of the hand.

Teeth

The reflexes for the front teeth are on the forefinger, and the side and back teeth range across the other fingers.

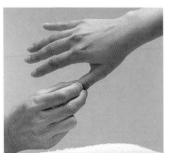
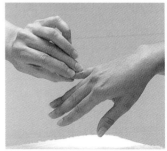

Eyes

The eye reflexes lie beneath the point where the second and third fingers meet the palm.

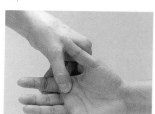

Sinuses

The reflex areas for the sinuses are located on the side of the fingers just below the first finger joint.

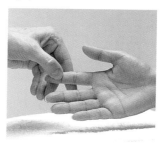

Ears

The ear reflexes lie beneath the junction with the fourth and fifth fingers, in the palm.

Eustachian tube

The Eustachian tube lies between the third and fourth fingers; it may sometimes be found in a similar position on the back of the hand.

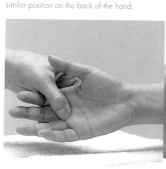

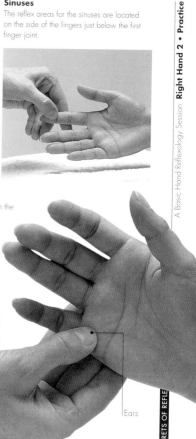

Ears

Right Hand 3 • Theory

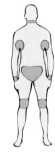

Vital organs
*Rebalancing the energy
in these areas can
improve well-being.*

As she continues to work the right hand, the reflexologist will treat all the reflexes as part of the treatment of the whole body, including those which are only found on this side. Among the most important of these are the reflex areas for the liver, the gallbladder, and the upper parts of the large intestine. If any of these organs is not working as well as it should be, the reflex areas may feel a little tender and the person may experience digestive problems and feel vaguely unwell. The person may also be prone to catching infections if the spleen, an important part of the immune system, is not doing its job properly: the white blood cells (lymphocytes) it produces help the body to fight off infection.

Lymphatics

The lymphatics are also important in tackling infectious organisms. Lymph nodes (or "glands") act as filters to trap bacteria and other foreign bodies. They are located in several important sites in the body, such as the neck, armpit, and groin, and each has its own small reflex area on the back of the hand. A fluid called lymph, which flows through the channels (or lymph vessels) linking the nodes, carries toxins and other waste products from the body's blood cells so that it can be purified in the nodes before being returned to the bloodstream. To encourage good drainage of lymph, the reflexologist will work a reflex just below where the base of the thumb joins the base of the forefinger on the back of the hand.

Injury

Hand treatment may be the favored option when there is a problem, such as an injury, which makes it impractical to treat the feet. So, an injury to the right hip or knee or symptoms of arthritis in these joints, for example, will be treated using the appropriate reflexes in the right hand. This may be appropriate when treating older people, in particular. Working these areas thoroughly will help to ease the pain and reduce any stiffness or lack of normal mobility.

Reproductive organs

In the hands, the reflexes for the male and female reproductive organs are found around the wrist area. Treating these is important in maintaining sexual health and function: it will help to restore the correct energy balance and may alleviate symptoms arising in these areas, such as menstrual difficulties in women and prostate problems in men, and stimulate fertility.

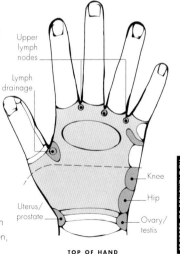

Upper lymph nodes

Lymph drainage

Knee

Hip

Uterus/ prostate

Ovary/ testis

TOP OF HAND

RIGHT HAND 3 • PRACTICE

The reflexes for the hip and knee, which also represent the upper and lower parts of the leg, are on the back of the hand. Immediately below the hip reflex, where the hand meets the wrist, is the reflex for the ovary/testis. Just before the wrist on the inner edge of the hand, are the reflexes for the uterus/prostate. The lymphatic system is represented on the back of the hand.

Knee

The knee reflex is close to the inside edge, below the little finger, about halfway between its base and the wrist.

Hip

The hip reflex is just below the knee reflex, closer to the wrist. It will also be treated if there are problems originating in the thigh.

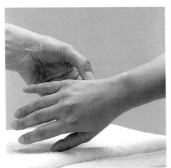

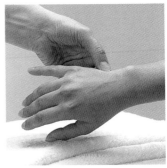

Uterus/prostate

The reflexes for a woman's uterus and a man's prostate gland extend from the palm around to the back of the hand.

Ovary/testis

This reflex, below the hip reflex, extends around the hand so that it is partly on the back and partly on the palm.

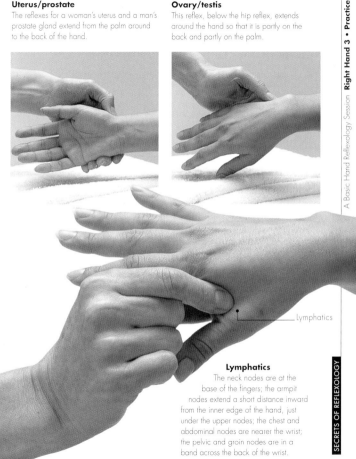

Lymphatics

Lymphatics

The neck nodes are at the base of the fingers; the armpit nodes extend a short distance inward from the inner edge of the hand, just under the upper nodes; the chest and abdominal nodes are nearer the wrist; the pelvic and groin nodes are in a band across the back of the wrist.

Left Hand • Theory

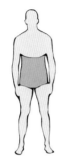

Unique reflexes
The heart and parts of the digestive system only appear on the left hand.

When the reflexologist moves onto the left hand she will work all the reflexes that were worked on the right hand in addition to reflexes that are only represented on this hand.

Heart

One of the most important reflexes which is represented on the left hand is that for the heart; it is found in zones 2 and 3 on the palm, about 1 inch (2.5 centimeters) down from the fingers. The heart reflex must be treated with great care, especially in anyone with a diagnosed heart condition, and it is important not to overwork this reflex. It is not suitable for self-treatment except under the direction of an experienced reflexologist. Correctly treated, however, it will help to promote a healthy circulation, which is vital to ensure that all parts of the body receive a good supply of oxygen and important nutrients carried in the bloodstream, and that toxins and other waste products such as carbon dioxide are removed effectively from the body.

Large intestine

As on the feet, the reflexes for the large intestine are divided between the left and right hands. The final parts of the digestive system extract the water needed by the body as the undigested component of the food the person has eaten passes through it. If the large intestine is not functioning correctly, the person may have problems such as constipation or diarrhea, and become dehydrated. The parts of the system represented on the left hand are the end of the transverse colon, the descending and sigmoid colons, and the rectum.

Kidneys

The kidneys extract a wide range of substances from the blood that passes through them, and transmit fluid not needed by the body to the bladder so that it can be passed out as urine. Treating these reflexes will help with infections, such as cystitis, and may help to ease urinary problems caused by prostate disease.

Adrenal glands

The two adrenal glands are positioned just above each of the kidneys, and produce a range of hormones which, among other things, stimulate the "fight-or-flight" response in a person facing a stressful situation, help to regulate the metabolism, and play a part in controlling the body's response to injury and allergens.

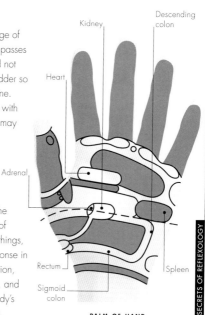

Kidney

Descending colon

Heart

Adrenal

Rectum

Sigmoid colon

Spleen

PALM OF HAND

LEFT HAND • PRACTICE

The reflexes for the heart and spleen are found in the palm of the left hand. The transverse colon reflex extends right across the palm, turning toward the wrist to form the reflex for the descending colon and then turning through a right angle again to represent the sigmoid colon. The reflex for the rectum is in zone 1.

Heart
The heart reflex is within zones 2 and 3 just above diaphragm level.

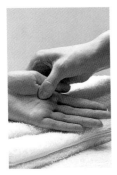

Spleen
The spleen is in zones 4 and 5, just above the waist line, in the left hand only.

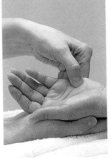

Kidney
The kidney is located on the palm in zones 2 and 3, around waist level.

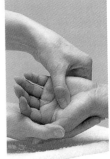

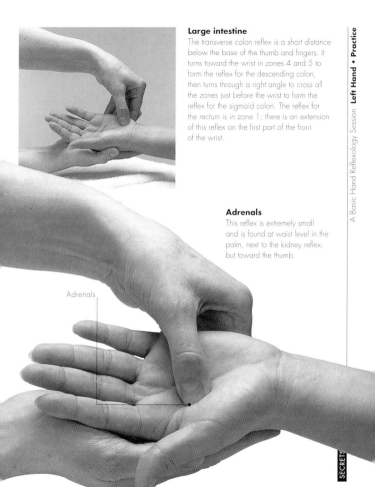

Large intestine

The transverse colon reflex is a short distance below the base of the thumb and fingers. It turns toward the wrist in zones 4 and 5 to form the reflex for the descending colon, then turns through a right angle to cross all the zones just before the wrist to form the reflex for the sigmoid colon. The reflex for the rectum is in zone 1; there is an extension of this reflex on the first part of the front of the wrist.

Adrenals

This reflex is extremely small and is found at waist level in the palm, next to the kidney reflex, but toward the thumb.

Adrenals

How to Treat
Your Own Hands

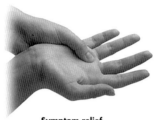

Symptom relief
*Treating your own hands
can be a useful form of
first aid.*

Although self-treatment on the hands
is not recommended as a
substitute for a full course of
treatment from a qualified practitioner,
it can be useful as a reinforcement
between sessions or to relieve specific
symptoms. You may choose to follow a
complete treatment as explained on the
previous pages, although this is difficult
to do when treating yourself; or to treat
a limited number of reflex areas related
to parts of your body that are currently
causing you problems.

Treatment

Choose a quiet place where you will
not be disturbed, and rest your right
hand on a cushion on your lap so that
it is at a comfortable and convenient
height to be worked with your other
hand. Spread a little talcum powder
over the skin on the hand you are
going to treat. Use the charts on pages
34–37 to locate the reflex points. The
small size of the hands means many
areas are extremely small, and you will
need to work with great precision.

In general, you will be using the top
of your thumb to apply pressure and you
will be able to adjust the level to what
feels right for you. Remember to keep
your thumb bent and avoid digging into
your skin with your nail. For awkward
areas, apply the same principle using
the top of your index finger.

Treat all the reflex points, giving extra
time to any areas that are tender or that
relate to a part of your body that you
know or sense is not working properly.

Once you have completed treatment on your right hand, do the same to your left hand, paying attention to any troublesome areas. Then do the hand relaxation exercises shown on the following pages. Of course, you will not be able to work both solar plexus reflexes simultaneously.

Self-treatment

Once you have learned the position of the appropriate reflex points on your hands, you will easily be able to treat symptoms such as a headache or back pain whenever or wherever you need to. This can be especially effective during a course of treatment from a reflexologist, which is focusing on such a recurring problem.

Relaxation

It is difficult to achieve a profound level of relaxation when treating yourself, so if you are tense and stressed, consider consulting a professional therapist.

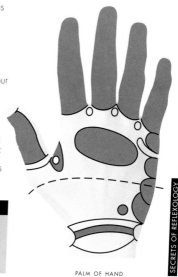

PALM OF HAND

HAND RELAXATION

Once the reflexologist has completed the basic treatment of both hands, she will complete the session with some relaxation exercises. As with the feet, these are done at the end of the session when the hands are already somewhat relaxed and more flexible, but they may sometimes also be done at the beginning of the session if the receiver (or her hands) are particularly tense.

Pressure

Different forms of pressure and movement are applied to the fingers and hands so as to stretch the related areas of the body and help the receiver to "wind down" after having a reflexology treatment.

Kneading

The therapist will knead the palm, using her fist, and will then rotate the wrists in both directions to dissolve any remaining obstacles to the free flow of energy through the body.

Rotation

In another technique known as "rotation," working first on the right hand and then on the left, the reflexologist will gently rotate each finger in turn in both directions. Then she will "wring" the palm.

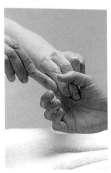

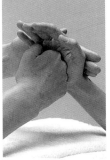

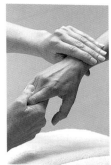

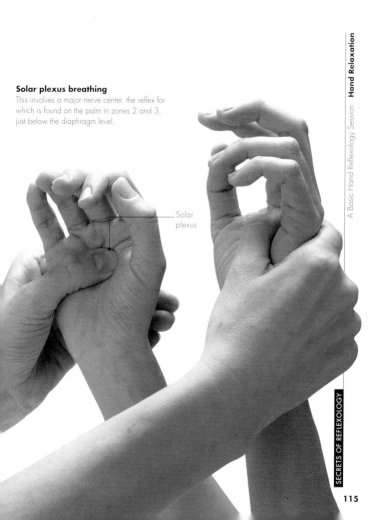

Solar plexus breathing

This involves a major nerve center, the reflex for which is found on the palm in zones 2 and 3, just below the diaphragm level.

Solar
plexus

Closing Down after Hand Reflexology

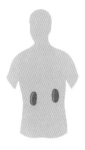

Excess toxins
As a side effect of reflexology the kidneys may work extra hard to excrete excess toxins.

The active part of the treatment is completed with an exercise called solar plexus breathing, which is designed to leave the receiver feeling calm and to round off the session in a peaceful way.

Solar plexus breathing

Working now on both hands at the same time, the therapist places her thumbs on the solar plexus reflex points on the palms, and supports the hands by placing her fingers on the backs. She then asks the receiver to take a deep breath, and as the air is inhaled she applies pressure with her thumbs while lifting the hands gently up toward the receiver's body. The receiver then breathes out, and, as she does so, the pressure is eased and her hands are lowered again.

Discussion and planning

As with a foot treatment, the final minutes of the reflexology session can be used by both giver and receiver to assess how the treatment has gone. The receiver can explain her perception—how she reacted while being treated and how she feels now it is complete. The reflexologist may point out any special areas of tenderness or other signs that certain parts of the body are not working as well as they should be, and can also recommend what further treatment might be beneficial.

Side effects

The therapist will also explain that, although everyone reacts differently in the period following treatment, minor side effects are not unusual, particularly slight feelings of nausea, a runny nose as the sinuses clear, and a need to visit the toilet more often than usual as toxins are excreted by the kidneys and bowels. Feeling energized and feeling tired are both common reactions but, like all the possible side effects, these should disappear within 48 hours or so. The fact that side effects, known as the "healing crisis" (see page 93), do develop is often regarded as a sign that the reflexology is having a beneficial effect, although not everyone who undergoes therapy experiences them.

Report Back

If you experience any severe or prolonged side effects, let your therapist know at your next session in case your treatment needs to be adjusted.

REFLEXOLOGY FOR HEALING

During a treatment session, all the reflex points will be worked, but special attention will be paid to areas that relate to symptoms arising in specific parts of the body. ☙ The reflexologist will take into account all aspects of the patient's life and personality, as well as any specific symptoms. By restoring the body's natural, healthy energy balance, treatment helps to stimulate and promote the body's innate ability to heal itself. ☙ Occasionally, treatment can be concentrated on particular reflexes to alleviate individual symptoms, or you can self-treat the areas, but better results will be obtained by incorporating symptomatic treatment in a full reflexology session. For complete maps of all the reflex areas see pages 30–37.

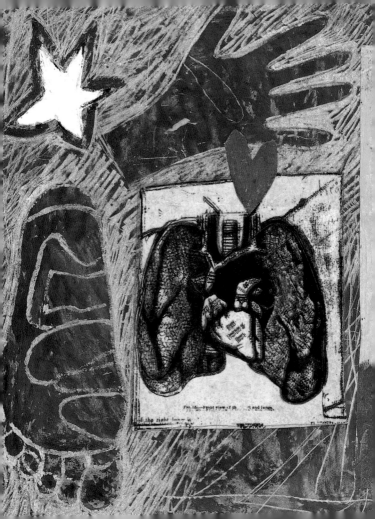

FIG. 33.—Front view of th... t and lungs.

...of the right lung i...

Respiratory Disorders

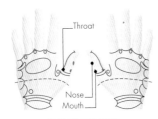

BACK OF THE HAND

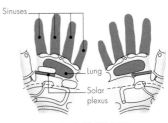

PALM OF THE HAND

Symptoms arising from problems affecting the respiratory system are extremely common, yet they can have a wide variety of causes and, with conditions such as asthma, may be exacerbated by other factors such as stress and lifestyle.

Causes

The majority of respiratory infections is caused by viruses, although sometimes bacteria may be involved. Antibiotics may have a useful part to play, but it is essential that these are not prescribed unless they are absolutely necessary. Asthmatics should continue taking their regular medication, although if a course of reflexology

treatment is successful, it may be possible to adjust the dosage if the patient's doctor agrees.

Asthma

The direct reflexes to be treated are those for the lungs and the bronchi—the hollow tubes that carry air to and from the trachea (the tube through which air passes to and from the lungs) and the lungs. Associated reflexes include the solar plexus and diaphragm, in order to promote relaxation; the cervical and thoracic spine, which represent the origin of the nerves supplying the bronchi and the lungs; and the adrenals, in order to treat stress and allergic reaction.

Colds

The direct reflexes to be treated are those for the nose and sinuses—the air-filled spaces in the skull bones; indirect reflexes that may also be treated are the adrenals, to reduce inflammation, and the upper lymph nodes, to help counteract infection.

Phlegm

The direct reflexes to be treated are the same as for colds, in addition to others, depending on whether the symptom is the result of infection (upper lymph nodes), or allergy (adrenals), or is associated with headache (head).

Coughs

The direct reflexes are the lungs and throat; the lymphatic system may also be treated to clear any infection.

Sinusitis

As well as the sinus reflexes, the face, nose, head, eyes, and ileocecal valve may be treated to ease congestion, eliminate mucus, and relieve pain.

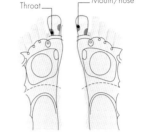

TOP OF THE FOOT

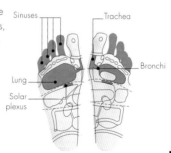

SOLE OF THE FOOT

TREATMENT ROUTINES

Respiratory disorders can affect all parts of the system—from the nose and sinuses to the trachea and the lungs themselves. As well as the directly related reflexes, the therapist will also treat those which are indirectly related—to reduce inflammation or help the immune system fight an infection, for example. The lymph nodes around the neck region are particularly important in dealing with a cold or other upper respiratory tract virus.

Colds

The reflex area for the nose is within that for the face, and is located just below the nail on the front of the big toe.

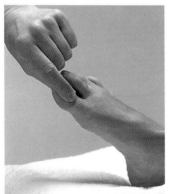

Sinusitis

The reflex areas for the sinuses are on the base and sides of the toes and the front and sides of the fingers.

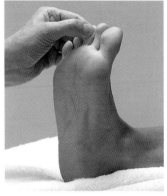

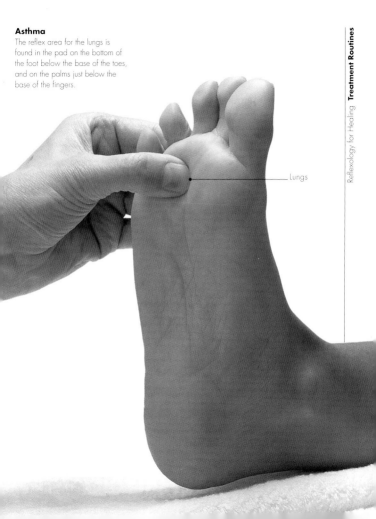

Asthma

The reflex area for the lungs is found in the pad on the bottom of the foot below the base of the toes, and on the palms just below the base of the fingers.

Lungs

Digestive Disorders

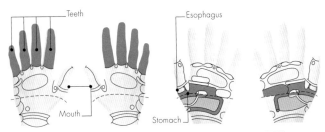

BACK OF THE HAND

Teeth

Mouth

PALM OF THE HAND

Esophagus

Stomach

Most of us experience digestive symptoms at some time, and generally regard them as no more than a relatively minor nuisance, especially when they have been brought on by something obvious like eating a very fatty or highly spiced meal. Nevertheless, symptoms that occur on a regular basis, or begin for the first time in a person in middle or later life, should be investigated by a doctor, since they may occasionally be the result of a serious condition that requires orthodox treatment. Usually such causes can be ruled out, however, and, more often than not, digestive problems are a consequence of stress or lifestyle factors such as smoking,

drinking too much alcohol, eating the wrong kind of food, or eating meals irregularly or in a rush.

Although there is no harm in taking the occasional over-the-counter remedy to settle troublesome symptoms, it makes much more sense to tackle the root cause of the problem, which is where reflexology can be very helpful, especially in cases of stress and tension.

Canker sores

Canker sores are usually insignificant from a medical point of view, but they can nevertheless be very painful and ruin your enjoyment of meals. Anyone who has frequent canker sores or ones that refuse to heal should have them

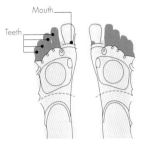

Mouth

Teeth

TOP OF THE FOOT

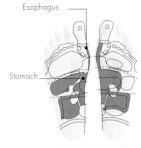

Esophagus

Stomach

SOLE OF THE FOOT

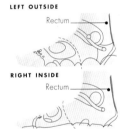

LEFT OUTSIDE

Rectum

RIGHT INSIDE

Rectum

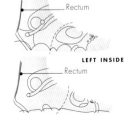

RIGHT OUTSIDE

Rectum

LEFT INSIDE

Rectum

checked out by their doctor or dentist to rule out other more serious conditions, but otherwise reflexology may help to promote the natural healing process.

Indigestion

Indigestion is usually the result of lifestyle factors, including diet and stress. During the initial consultation, the reflexologist will discuss how you can change aspects of your life that might be the underlying cause of your symptoms. As for treatment, the main direct reflex area is the stomach, but if the symptoms include heartburn, the reflex areas for the esophagus and diaphragm will also be treated. (See also Diarrhea and Constipation on pages 132–135.)

TREATMENT ROUTINES

The reflexologist's aim is to ease pain and encourage the body's natural ability to heal itself by unblocking energy flow and restoring a proper balance. For canker sores, the reflex areas to be treated are those for the face, teeth, and upper lymphatics. Treatment for symptoms relating to the esophagus and stomach involves the reflex areas for the esophagus, stomach, solar plexus, and diaphragm, plus the adrenals.

Mouth

Reflex areas for the face are on the front of the big toes, and the top of the thumbs, below the nails. They are relatively small and thus treatment must be extremely precise in order to target the right areas.

Esophagus

The esophagus reflex on the feet is down the inner edge of the sole from just below the big toe to the level of the diaphragm. On the hand it is toward the edge of the palm, above where the thumb joins the hand.

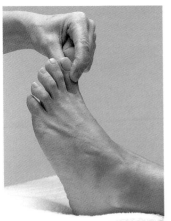

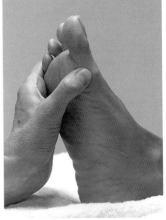

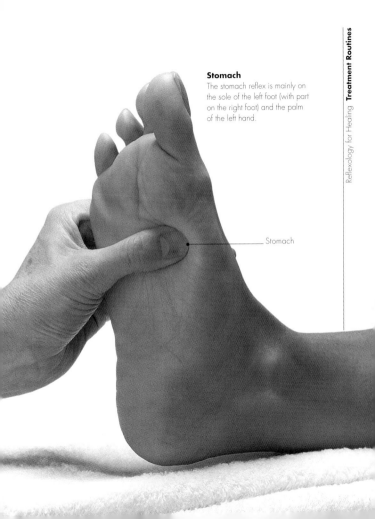

Stomach

The stomach reflex is mainly on the sole of the left foot (with part on the right foot) and the palm of the left hand.

Stomach

Liver and Gallbladder Disorders

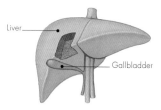

Liver

Gallbladder

The liver
This is one of the most important organs in the whole body.

The liver and gallbladder are key components of metabolism, the means by which food is processed so that it can be used to fuel and to maintain all bodily functions.

Functions

The liver controls many essential chemical reactions, including the storage and release of glucose and of important minerals and vitamins, and the breakdown of fats, alcohol, and other toxins. A thick, green fluid, called bile, is made in the liver and passed for storage to the gallbladder. From there, it will be released into the intestines when needed to break up digested fat into tiny globules which can be absorbed into the bloodstream.

Disorders

Any disorder that interferes with the proper working of either of these organs needs investigation by orthodox doctors and, almost invariably, conventional treatment with drugs, surgery, or both. Liver disease—of which the first sign is often jaundice—is potentially very serious and can be fatal if it is left untreated. Poor fat digestion may occur if the gallbladder is not functioning properly, resulting in abdominal discomfort and pale, offensive stools.

Recovery

Once the cause of any symptoms has been diagnosed, and any necessary orthodox treatment has been started (or completed), a reflexology treatment can play a truly complementary role in speeding up recovery and easing any symptoms that remain. It can also help to treat less serious symptoms that may be the result of imbalances, which prevent these important organs from working as well as they should.

Regeneration

The liver is capable of regenerating damaged areas once the underlying cause of the damage has been dealt with, provided that the problem is diagnosed and treated in time. Reflexology treatment may be helpful following conventional treatment of liver disorders by encouraging the body's natural ability to heal itself.

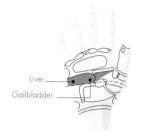

PALM OF THE RIGHT HAND

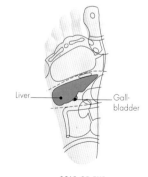

SOLE OF THE RIGHT FOOT

Gallstones

Severe pain on the right side in the upper abdomen may be a sign of gallstones—hard lumps made up of cholesterol, bile pigments, and calcium salts that sometimes form within the gallbladder.

TREATMENT ROUTINES

The reflex areas to be treated in cases of poor fat digestion are the liver, gallbladder, and stomach. For jaundice, which is often a sign of liver disease, the liver, gallbladder, and the reflex areas for the relevant lymphatics will be treated. Gallstones are treated by manipulation of the gallbladder, liver, and solar plexus reflexes.

Poor fat digestion

The reflex area is the gallbladder, in zone 3 of the right foot and hand only, just above waist level. The stomach reflex, mainly on the left foot and hand, may also need treating.

Jaundice

The liver reflex is found only on the right foot and hand, stretching across all five zones on the sole and on the palm between the diaphragm and waist levels.

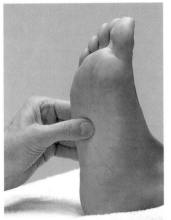

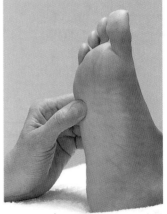

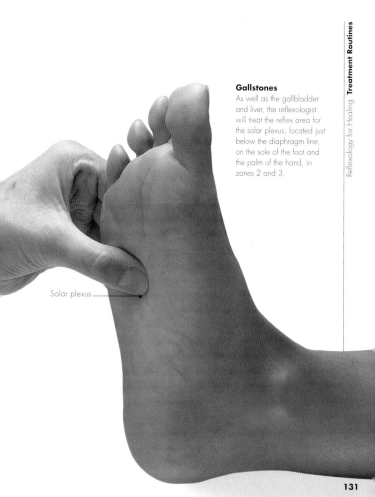

Gallstones

As well as the gallbladder and liver, the reflexologist will treat the reflex area for the solar plexus, located just below the diaphragm line, on the sole of the foot and the palm of the hand, in zones 2 and 3.

Solar plexus

Diarrhea and Constipation

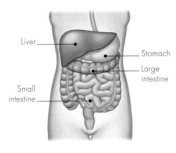

The digestive process
Enzymes produced by the digestive organs break down our food.

Liver
Stomach
Large intestine
Small intestine

If you develop either (or both) of these symptoms for the first time and they last longer than a few days or recur often, you should consult your doctor; diarrhea and constipation can be associated with serious conditions, such as ulcerative colitis, Crohn's disease, or occasionally cancer. You should also tell your doctor if you have been abroad to any country where you might have contracted an infection or other illness—such as typhoid—rarely encountered at home. Symptoms that only last a couple of days are more likely to have a

dietary cause or, in the case of diarrhea, be the result of a mild form of food poisoning or a slight infection, and will disappear without treatment.

Irritable bowel syndrome

Irritable bowel syndrome (IBS) is a particularly difficult condition which can cause both diarrhea and constipation. It is often made worse by stress and anxiety, and results from irregular peristalsis, the wavelike action of the intestine that propels feces toward the rectum. There is no obvious cause and IBS can abate for long periods. Treatment requires work on the reflex areas for the large intestine, liver, adrenals, and solar plexus.

Diarrhea

The direct reflex to be treated is the large intestine, which is passing the products of digestion through too fast before the water content can be absorbed properly, which can lead to dehydration. If the cause of diarrhea is an infection, the abdominal lymphatics

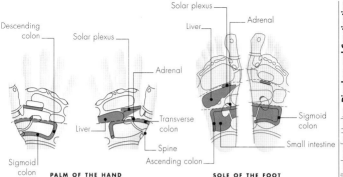

Descending colon
Solar plexus
Adrenal
Liver
Transverse colon
Spine
Sigmoid colon

PALM OF THE HAND

Solar plexus
Adrenal
Liver
Sigmoid colon
Small intestine
Ascending colon

SOLE OF THE FOOT

reflex area will also be treated. The solar plexus and adrenals will be treated to promote relaxation and the small intestine may also require treatment.

Constipation

Treatment for constipation is needed for the sluggish bowel in the ascending and sigmoid colon areas, but several associated reflex areas will also be worked, including the small intestine, liver, the adrenals, and those in the lower spine.

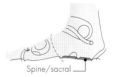

Spine/sacral

RIGHT INSIDE

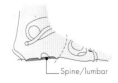

Spine/lumbar

LEFT INSIDE

Lifestyle

If symptoms of diarrhea and/or constipation persist, despite your doctor being unable to find any specific cause, they are likely to be related to lifestyle factors.

TREATMENT ROUTINES
After a discussion on relevant aspects of the person's lifestyle, especially diet and stress, the reflexologist will need to work on a number of reflex areas when treating either of these conditions. Diarrhea requires treatment of various parts of the large intestine. Associated reflex areas are the abdominal lymphatics, solar plexus, adrenals, and small intestine. Constipation requires work on parts of the large intestine, small intestine, liver, the adrenals, and the solar plexus.

Large intestine
Surrounding the area for the small intestine is the reflex area for the large intestine, which is made up of several sections, some on the right foot (or hand) and some on the left. The ascending colon and part of the transverse colon are on the right foot (and hand); the remainder of the transverse colon, the descending and sigmoid colons, and the rectum are on the left side.

Small intestine
The reflex area for the small intestine is found on the soles of both feet, just above the heel pad across zones 1 to 4. On the hand, it is located on the palm, between the waist level and the wrist across the same zones.

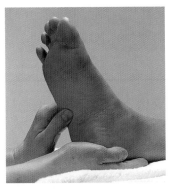

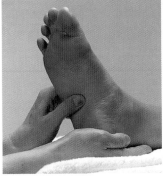

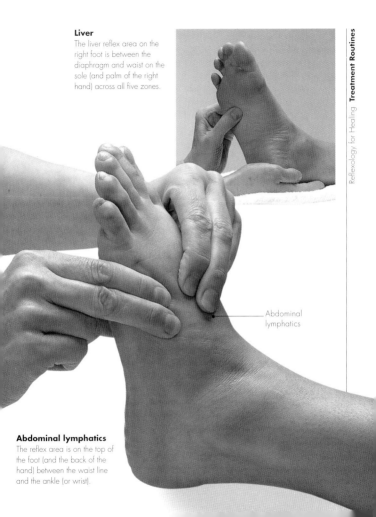

Liver

The liver reflex area on the right foot is between the diaphragm and waist on the sole (and palm of the right hand) across all five zones.

Abdominal lymphatics

Abdominal lymphatics

The reflex area is on the top of the foot (and the back of the hand) between the waist line and the ankle (or wrist).

Heart and Circulation Disorders

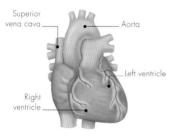

The heart
The heart pumps oxygenated blood around the body.

- Superior vena cava
- Aorta
- Left ventricle
- Right ventricle

Reflexology treatment should be given to a person with a heart condition only by an experienced reflexologist, and then with great care. However, reflexology can be very beneficial in conditions in which poor circulation is a factor, such as angina, palpitations, cold extremities, and varicose veins. It can also play an important part in maintaining a healthy circulation: efficient blood flow is vital because it carries oxygen and other vital nutrients via the arteries to every cell in the body, and removes waste products and toxins. Reflex work to optimize heart function and improve circulation will form part of a full treatment in all cases, and extra attention will be paid to the left hand and foot, where the reflex area for the heart is located.

Angina

Angina results in pain in the chest area whenever the body's demands for oxygen rise—when walking upstairs, for example, and often comes on in cold, windy weather. It is caused by a narrowing of the blood vessels near the heart, which restricts the free flow of blood, but the symptoms respond well to conventional medication.

Palpitations

Palpitations—irregular heartbeats—need to be investigated properly, but often no underlying cause can be found. Reflexology may relieve the problem by alleviating stress and improving the body's energy balance.

Poor circulation

Poor circulation can result in other symptoms which, although not serious, are unpleasant. Varicose veins most commonly appear in the lower legs or vulva during pregnancy. Poor circulation in the hands or feet can leave them vulnerable to cold and they may look very pale or even bluish. The same reflex areas will be treated for cold extremities and varicose veins, including the heart, small and large intestines, spine, and the zone-related areas for the part of the body affected.

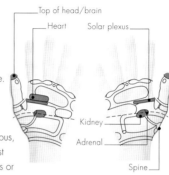

PALM OF THE HAND

Chilblains

Poor circulation may cause red, itchy swellings—chilblains—to develop, mostly on the toes, in damp, cold weather, particularly when the blood vessels react inappropriately to cold.

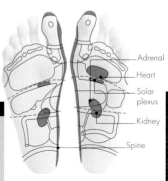

SOLE OF THE FOOT

TREATMENT ROUTINES

Reflexology treatment to stimulate the circulation and dispel energy blockages can be beneficial in any condition related to the heart and circulation. The heart, solar plexus, and adrenals reflex areas treat both angina and palpitations. Sluggish circulation is treated by the heart, small and large intestines, spine, and zone-related areas. Treatment of the adrenals reflex areas may help lower blood pressure, but should not be considered as an alternative to any prescribed medication.

Angina

The reflex area for the heart is found only on the left foot and left hand. In the foot, it is just above diaphragm level in the lower part of the ball, and in the palm of the hand it is in zones 2 and 3, just above diaphragm level.

Palpitations

The solar plexus is the most appropriate reflex area to treat, found just below diaphragm level, in zones 2 and 3, in the sole of the foot and approximately one-quarter of the distance down the palm from the fingers.

High blood pressure

High blood pressure is treated by pressure on the adrenals, small areas found just above waist level on the soles and palms, toward the inner edges of the feet and hands.

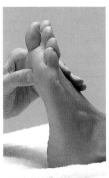

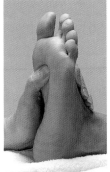

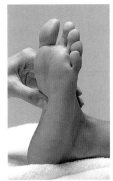

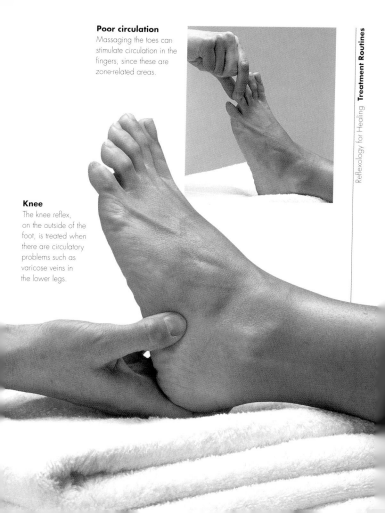

Poor circulation
Massaging the toes can stimulate circulation in the fingers, since these are zone-related areas.

Knee
The knee reflex, on the outside of the foot, is treated when there are circulatory problems such as varicose veins in the lower legs.

The Lymphatic System

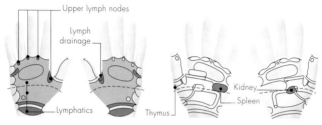

BACK OF THE HAND

Upper lymph nodes

Lymph drainage

Lymphatics

PALM OF THE HAND

Kidney

Spleen

Thymus

The lymphatic system is part of the extremely complex and all-important immune system, which defends the body against illness and acts as a "drainage" system through which the body can expel various toxins and waste products. The lymphatic system consists of a network of hollow vessels with a structure similar to that of the circulatory system. These carry lymph, a pale yellow fluid, which nourishes the tissue cells and removes their waste products. Lymph nodes (or "glands") are located at key points throughout the system, where they function as filters to trap invading organisms such as bacteria. They also manufacture some of the white blood cells, called lymphocytes, which are responsible for the production of antibodies that fight foreign bodies.

Problems

A number of factors can weaken the immune system and inhibit its effectiveness, including infections, prolonged stress, immunosuppressant drugs, and conditions such as chronic fatigue, HIV, and AIDS. In such circumstances, a vicious circle can develop in which the body is unable to fight off other infections or illnesses, which in turn reduces the effectiveness of the immune system still further. Fluid retention is often a symptom of PMS and can cause swollen ankles in later pregnancy.

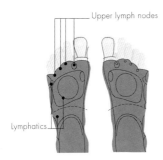

TOP OF THE FOOT

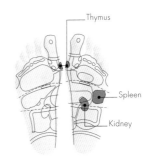

SOLE OF THE FOOT

Swollen nodes

As most of us know from experience, the lymph nodes swell when nearby tissue is under attack: this is why the "glands" in your neck below your ears enlarge and become tender when you have a bad throat infection, for example. This is part of the attempt by the body's immune system to contain an infection and prevent the organisms responsible from spreading throughout the rest of the body.

Depleted Immune System

Stress and emotional, dietary, and lifestyle factors all put strain on the immune system. Excessive exercise, lack of sleep, and smoking may also overload the system.

LEFT OUTSIDE

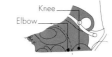

RIGHT INSIDE

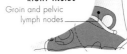

RIGHT OUTSIDE

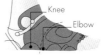

LEFT INSIDE

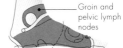

TREATMENT ROUTINES
The main reflex areas for fluid retention are the kidneys, but the lymphatics, the ureter tubes, the bladder, pituitary, heart, liver, and the area affected may also be treated. In cases of poor immune function, the reflex areas for the lymphatic system will be treated. Since swollen "glands" are actually lymph nodes, the reflex areas for the affected nodes will need to be treated, as will the spleen.

Fluid retention

The kidney reflexes are located on the sole of the foot and on the palm, at waist level in zones 2 and 3. They will be treated in order to improve the body's ability to excrete urine and thus alleviate fluid retention.

Poor immune function

The reflex for the spleen, which is an important part of the immune system, is only on the left foot and hand. It is found on the sole and palm in zones 4 and 5 between the diaphragm and the waist.

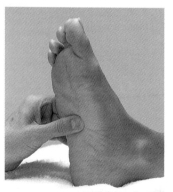

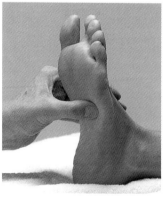

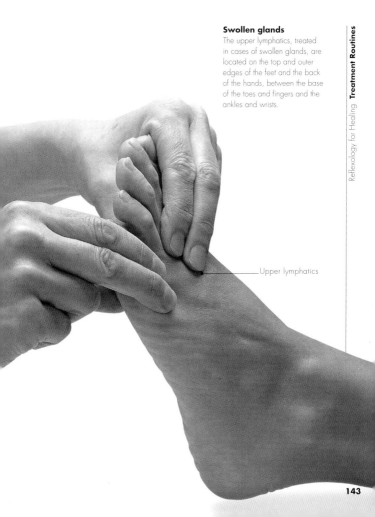

Swollen glands

The upper lymphatics, treated in cases of swollen glands, are located on the top and outer edges of the feet and the back of the hands, between the base of the toes and fingers and the ankles and wrists.

Upper lymphatics

Urinary Disorders

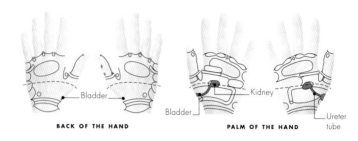

BACK OF THE HAND

PALM OF THE HAND

Pain or other problems associated with the urinary tract can have a variety of causes, but probably the most common is an infection of some kind. Infectious organisms enter through the urethra (the tube through which urine is eliminated) and can then spread to the bladder and beyond to the kidneys.

Cystitis

Bladder infection (cystitis) is more common in women because the urethra is much shorter and located closer to the anus than it is in men, and this is one source of potential bacterial infection. Once an infection has become established, it can be difficult to treat, although antibiotics may be effective in some cases. If the first course of prescribed antibiotics does not cure the condition, it may be necessary to test a urine sample to establish exactly which bacteria are present. Drinking lots of water may help to ease the pain and cranberry juice can also help to relieve symptoms. A reflexologist will treat the bladder and associated organs and will work to improve the efficiency of the immune system (see pages 140–143) to make a recurrence less likely.

Bladder problems

In later life, many men start to have difficulty emptying their bladder as a result of enlargement of the prostate, which then compresses the urethra and stops the urine flowing freely. If the bladder also becomes squashed, cystitis may set in and the man may experience pain as well as problems urinating (see pages 212–213). Always consult your doctor if you experience difficulty passing urine.

Having to empty the bladder frequently is a normal side effect of pregnancy, again because of pressure on the bladder. Some women have trouble with leakage after giving birth because of damage to the pelvic floor muscles, which control the flow of urine. However, the need to empty the bladder very frequently needs to be investigated in anyone else, because it may be a symptom of a condition that needs medical treatment; diabetes being probably the most common disorder (see pages 148–149).

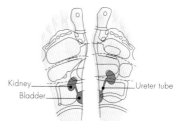

Kidney
Bladder
Ureter tube

SOLE OF THE FOOT

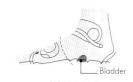

Bladder

RIGHT INSIDE

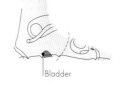

Bladder

LEFT INSIDE

Bacterial Infections

Bacterial infections of the urinary system, such as nonspecific urethritis (NSU), can cause pain upon urination and should be treated with a course of antibiotics.

TREATMENT ROUTINES

Most of the disorders associated with the urinary tract are caused by bacterial infections, although prostate enlargement, and pregnancy and its aftermath can cause bladder problems. Bladder infections require treatment of the bladder, kidneys, ureter, and pelvic lymphatics. The same areas will need to be treated for poor kidney function, with the addition of adrenals, pituitary, and parathyroid reflex areas. The treatment for prostate problems is explained on pages 212–213.

Bladder infections

The bladder reflex is located on the inner side of the foot just in front of the ankle bone and on the inside of the hand just above the wrist.

Poor kidney function

The kidney reflexes are found at waist level on the sole of the foot and the palm in zones 2 and 3.

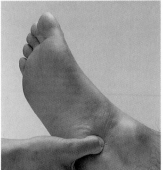

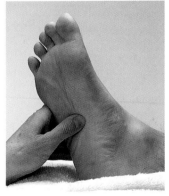

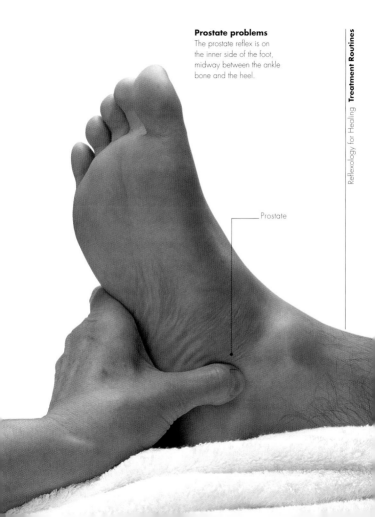

Prostate problems
The prostate reflex is on the inner side of the foot, midway between the ankle bone and the heel.

Prostate

Hormonal Disorders

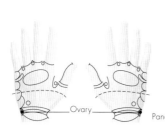

BACK OF THE HAND

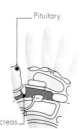

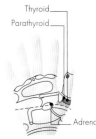

PALM OF THE HAND

Good physical and mental health depend on the body's ability to adjust the levels of "chemical messengers," called hormones, which are responsible for regulating a wide range of functions.

Action of hormones

Hormones are produced by a series of endocrine glands around the body, under the overall control of the pituitary gland at the base of the skull. When the system is working well, the pituitary triggers the release of individual hormones—and inhibits them when necessary—either according to the needs of the body at a particular moment, or on a cyclical basis. For

example, the adrenal glands, located just above the kidneys, release epinephrine and norepinephrine to enable the body to divert all the necessary resources to dealing with a threatening situation, either by "fight" or "flight." Other hormones, such as the growth hormone, or melatonin (the sleep hormone), are secreted at regular intervals, determined by the body's internal "clock." This delicate balancing act can become disrupted easily in a number of ways.

Apart from problems associated with the female hormones estrogen and progesterone (see pages 152–153), the most common conditions caused by hormone disruption are diabetes and thyroid disease. Both conditions need to be treated with orthodox medicine, but an experienced reflexologist can complement its effectiveness.

Diabetes

This develops when the pancreas stops releasing the hormone insulin, which is needed to absorb energy from food, or when the body becomes unable to respond to insulin properly. Type 1 (or insulin-dependent diabetes) usually begins relatively early in life as insulin production fails, but Type II (noninsulin-dependent diabetes) mostly affects people in middle or later years and is often treated with tablets and/or diet rather than with insulin injections.

Thyroid disease

The thyroid gland is found in the front of the neck and malfunction can cause a wide range of unpleasant symptoms. The most common is the over- or under-production of the hormone thyroxine, which controls metabolism. Orthodox treatment is relatively effective.

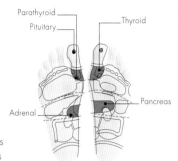

SOLE OF THE FOOT

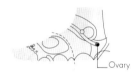

LEFT OUTSIDE

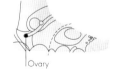

RIGHT OUTSIDE

TREATMENT ROUTINES

Reflexology treatment can complement orthodox therapy or may help to correct any minor imbalances that are causing the thyroid gland to work less well than it should, whether the problem is over- or underactivity. People with diabetes who are taking medication should be treated only by an experienced reflexologist. Other reflex areas may be treated if the person has symptoms affecting the heart, eyes, or kidneys, for example.

Thyroid
The thyroid reflex area is over the ball of the foot, just below the big toe, and in the palm of the hand just below the point where the thumb meets the hand.

Pituitary
The reflex area for the pituitary gland is located on the sole of the foot in the center of the fleshy pad on the underside of the big toe, and, on the palm, on the pad of the thumb.

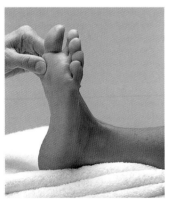

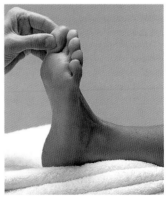

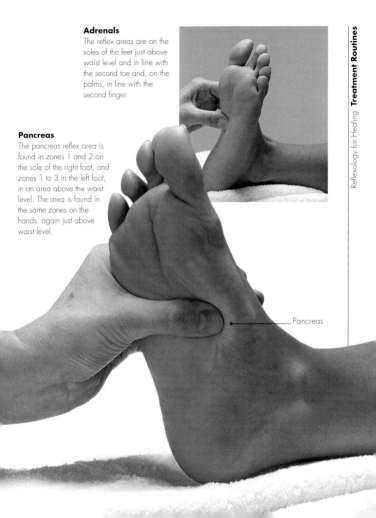

Adrenals
The reflex areas are on the soles of the feet just above waist level and in line with the second toe and, on the palms, in line with the second finger.

Pancreas
The pancreas reflex area is found in zones 1 and 2 on the sole of the right foot, and zones 1 to 3 in the left foot, in an area above the waist level. The area is found in the same zones on the hands, again just above waist level.

Pancreas

Reproductive System Disorders

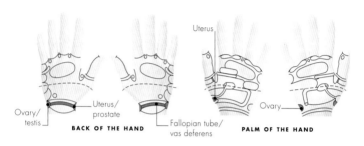

Ovary/testis | Uterus/prostate

BACK OF THE HAND

Uterus | Ovary | Fallopian tube/vas deferens

PALM OF THE HAND

Symptoms associated with a woman's menstrual cycle are so common as to be regarded as more or less normal, yet they are often distressing and disruptive of normal living. Such symptoms include premenstrual syndrome, painful and/or heavy periods, irregular or scanty periods, failure to conceive, and difficulties associated with the onset of menopause. Men are not subject to the same complex hormonal influences and so experience fewer symptoms than women, although they may have problems with infertility. They may also have difficulty achieving or sustaining an erection, a distressing problem that may be physiological or psychological in origin, or both.

Menstrual disorders

Menstrually-related symptoms are often the result of hormone imbalance, but can also be a sign that something is wrong with a particular part of the reproductive system. For example, painful, heavy periods can be caused by fibroids (benign growths in the uterus), endometriosis, when parts of the uterine lining migrate within the pelvis and bleed during menstruation, or pelvic inflammatory disease.

Infertility

Many factors, affecting either or both partners, can result in infertility, and tests will be needed to establish the cause and whether orthodox treatment is appropriate. Stress and tension may be playing a part, and reflexology can be very beneficial when treatment is given, not only for any underlying disorder, but also to promote relaxation.

The therapist will also give additional treatment to the reflex areas for the specific part or parts of the body that are not working properly. In women, this is likely to include the ovaries, uterus, and Fallopian tubes, as well as the pituitary and the abdominal area. The solar plexus will be treated to promote relaxation and dispel anxiety.

Treating Male Disorders

Treatment to the testes reflexes may help sperm production. Treatments to reduce anxiety and promote relaxation may also be effective.

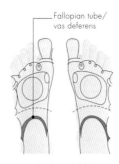

Fallopian tube/ vas deferens

TOP OF THE FOOT

LEFT OUTSIDE

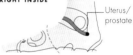

Ovary/ testis

RIGHT INSIDE

Uterus/ prostate

RIGHT OUTSIDE

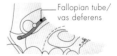

Fallopian tube/ vas deferens

LEFT INSIDE

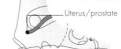

Uterus/prostate

TREATMENT ROUTINES

During treatment, extra attention will be given to the areas relating to the various parts of a woman's reproductive system and to the glands that regulate the hormonal system. Male infertility or lack of sex drive will be treated by focusing on the equivalent reproductive organs: the testes in the same areas as the ovaries, the vas deferens in the same area as the Fallopian tubes, and the prostate in the same area as the uterus.

Menstrual problems

The uterus reflex is at the same level as the ovaries on the inner edge of the foot; and in a similar position to the ovaries on the inner side of the hand.

Fertility problems

The Fallopian tubes reflex is located along a strip linking the ovaries and uterus across the top of the foot (and also across the back of the hand).

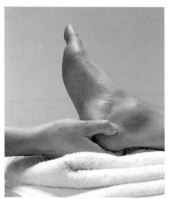

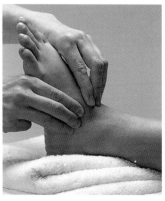

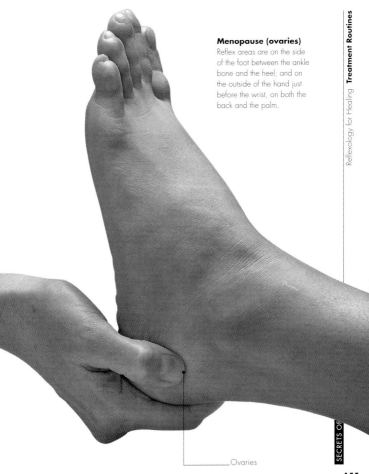

Menopause (ovaries)

Reflex areas are on the side of the foot between the ankle bone and the heel; and on the outside of the hand just before the wrist, on both the back and the palm.

Ovaries

Headaches and Migraines

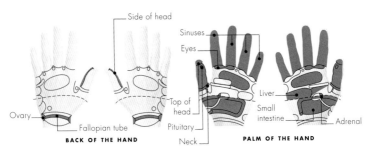

Side of head

Sinuses

Eyes

Ovary

Fallopian tube

Top of head

Liver

Small intestine

Adrenal

Pituitary

Neck

BACK OF THE HAND

PALM OF THE HAND

A headache can be just one symptom of an enormous range of conditions, a few of them serious, but most people get them at some time without there being any major underlying cause. Frequent, persistent, and disabling headaches should be investigated by a doctor, particularly in someone who has never suffered from them in the past. You would be wise to report a sudden, intense headache that comes out of the blue to your doctor; this can, on occasion, be a sign of a more serious problem. However, the vast majority of headaches are triggered by a minor viral infection, by physical or mental tension, or by migraines—when they may well be accompanied by other symptoms such as visual disturbance and nausea and, sometimes, vomiting.

Treatment

When possible, it is desirable to treat the root cause of the headache, rather than simply alleviating the pain. However, it is not always possible to identify this, and with migraines, the actual cause is not yet fully understood, although many migraine sufferers are well aware of what triggers them.

Reflex areas

While the head area will be treated as part of a reflexology session, other areas will also need to be worked

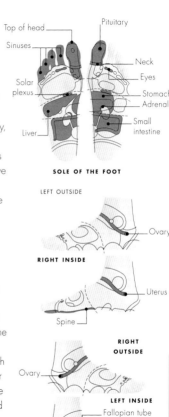

on, depending on the cause of the headache or associated symptoms. Treating the solar plexus and possibly the adrenals is important when the headache is related to stress or anxiety, and the neck, shoulders, and upper spine may also need treatment if stress is causing muscular tension. If you have a viral infection, the lymph nodes will be treated, and the sinuses if these are congested or inflamed.

Migraines

Migraines result from spasm and dilation of the arteries and blood vessels supplying the brain, causing a blinding headache with intense pain. This often causes additional symptoms and the reflexes for affected parts of the body will be treated as necessary. These reflexes may include the stomach (for nausea and sickness), the eyes (for visual disturbance), the small and large intestines (for an allergic reaction), and the pituitary and ovaries, if hormonal factors are involved and in cases of menstrual migraine.

SOLE OF THE FOOT

LEFT OUTSIDE

Ovary

RIGHT INSIDE

Uterus

Spine

RIGHT OUTSIDE

Ovary

LEFT INSIDE

Fallopian tube

Uterus

TREATMENT ROUTINES

The reflexologist will aim not only to ease and prevent the recurrence of headache and migraine symptoms, but also to treat those areas of the body that are responsible for triggering the symptoms in the first place. This will require careful assessment before treatment begins because there may be imbalances and stresses in several different areas, or the person may experience headaches from a number of distinct causes.

Head

The head reflexes are on the top, outer side, and underside of the big toe, and relate to the skull and the brain itself. In the hand, the reflex areas are around the top, the underside, and the side of the thumb next to the forefinger.

Neck

The reflexes for the front and back of the neck are located on the top and underneath of the base of the big toe and the thumb.

Spine

The cervical vertebrae are located along the inner edges of the big toe and the thumb. They will be treated if the neck and shoulders are tense.

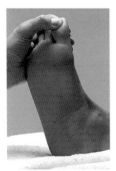

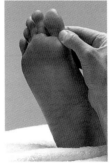

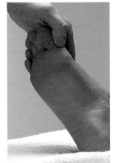

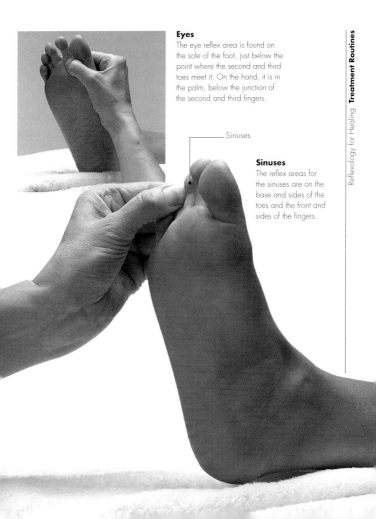

Eyes
The eye reflex area is found on the sole of the foot, just below the point where the second and third toes meet it. On the hand, it is in the palm, below the junction of the second and third fingers.

Sinuses

Sinuses
The reflex areas for the sinuses are on the base and sides of the toes and the front and sides of the fingers.

Anxiety and Depression

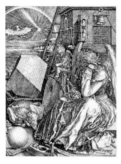

Depression
*This should not be
dismissed as being of
no consequence.*

Periods of feeling anxious or down in the dumps are a normal part of life for all but the most fortunate, but there is a very real difference between feeling bad for a day or two and feeling constantly weighed down or incapacitated by anxiety or depression. Constant, unfocused anxiety can limit your ability to live a normal life, and is often associated with other symptoms such as poor digestion and sleep, and headaches. Depression can be just as much a "real" illness as heart disease, for example, and you can no more snap out of it than you could out of a recognized physical condition.

Seek help

If you are affected by either of these conditions in a way which disrupts your life for more than a few days, do not be embarrassed to ask for professional help. Your doctor may suggest medication and/or some form of psychological therapy, which can both improve your mood and begin to deal with whatever is causing the symptoms. It is a mistake to regard such symptoms as a sign of weakness or a character flaw, and equally wrong to believe that you must just cope as best you can. Recovery may take time, but most people do get well again with the right kind of treatment. Try to follow a sensible and nutritious diet and resist the urge to turn to drugs or alcohol to alleviate your mood. Keeping yourself mentally and physically active may help to overcome some of your feelings.

Benefits of reflexology

Reflexology can play a significant part in helping you to feel better. As well as treating the direct reflex areas of the head and brain, the therapist will also work on associated areas, such as the adrenals (for anxiety), the pituitary and other endocrine glands (for hormonal imbalances), and the solar plexus for thorough relaxation.

Apart from the direct benefits of treatment to restore the body to good working order and correcting energy imbalances, many people find it helps to be free to express how they feel to a professional who is interested in all aspects of their life. The reflexologist will be prepared for the possibility that treatment may trigger emotional outbursts as the underlying tensions and problems surface.

Seasonal Affective Disorder

In the winter, many people experience a form of depression caused by a lack of light. Therapies such as reflexology that aid relaxation and improve well-being will help.

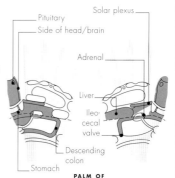

PALM OF THE HAND

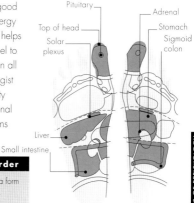

SOLE OF THE FOOT

TREATMENT ROUTINES

A course of treatment of the whole body will have a beneficial effect on general well-being, encouraging relaxation and restoring the body's energy balance in a secure and positive environment. The reflexologist will pay special attention to the reflex areas associated with individual symptoms. Correcting any imbalances in the hormonal and digestive systems may help to ease symptoms, and treating the solar plexus reflex is particularly important to encourage relaxation and relieve anxiety.

Solar plexus
The solar plexus reflex is found in the middle of the sole, just below the ball of the foot, and in the palm of the hand, in zones 2 and 3.

Adrenals
The adrenals are small areas which are located just above waist level on the soles and palms, toward the inner edges of the feet and hands.

Pituitary
The pituitary gland, which is located in the center of the base of the big toes, or thumbs, is treated to promote a healthy hormone balance.

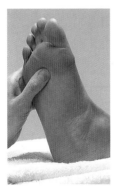
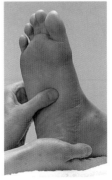
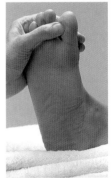

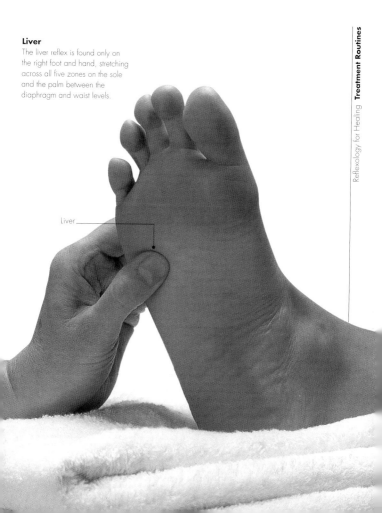

Liver
The liver reflex is found only on the right foot and hand, stretching across all five zones on the sole and the palm between the diaphragm and waist levels.

Liver

Sleeping Difficulties

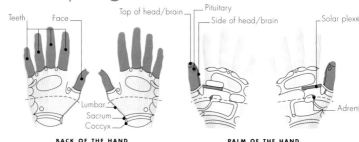

Teeth Face Top of head/brain Pituitary Side of head/brain Solar plexus

Lumbar
Sacrum
Coccyx

Adrenal

BACK OF THE HAND **PALM OF THE HAND**

One of the main problems with insomnia is that a vicious circle often develops: you worry that you are not sleeping well and the worry makes the sleeplessness worse. Most sleeping difficulties are not a symptom of a serious illness, and lack of sleep in itself will not do you any real harm. However, it will leave you feeling tired and irritable and make it hard to concentrate. It may also be dangerous if you drive or operate machinery while suffering from lack of sleep.

Solutions

If your inability to get a good night's sleep is related to symptoms of a specific condition—such as the pain of

arthritis, or depression—you should make sure you are getting the appropriate treatment from your doctor. You can also take some steps to make restful sleep more likely, including not eating a heavy meal late at night, resisting drinks containing caffeine in the evening, getting regular exercise, and avoiding too much mental stimulation as bedtime approaches. You should also try to ensure that your bed is comfortable and that the room is dark, quiet, and at the right temperature.

Mental relaxation

Reflexology for sleeping difficulties will aim to promote mental relaxation by treating the head and brain, and

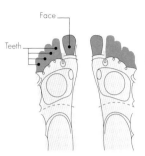

TOP OF THE FOOT

Face

Teeth

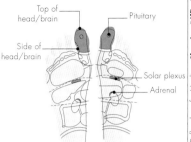

SOLE OF THE FOOT

Top of head/brain

Pituitary

Side of head/brain

Solar plexus

Adrenal

associated reflexes, such as the adrenals to combat stress, and those related to symptoms such as back or joint pain will also need extra attention. The overall rebalancing of the body's energy flow will also help to promote a good night's sleep, and many people also find it helps just having the opportunity to talk about any worries that are interfering with their sleep. It is worth trying this approach in preference to drug treatment.

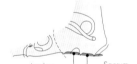

RIGHT INSIDE

Lumbar

Sacrum

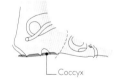

LEFT INSIDE

Coccyx

The Right Amount of Sleep

The amount of sleep we need depends on the individual and decreases as we get older. Research is contradictory but would indicate that six hours is the minimum we require.

TREATMENT ROUTINES

It is important to check with your doctor if you suspect sleeping difficulties may be associated with any condition that might need investigation and conventional treatment, such as arthritis or other painful illnesses, depression, or breathing difficulties. People who are depressed often find they wake very early and cannot get back to sleep, while anxiety and stress can make it difficult to get to sleep or cause frequent night waking.

Head/brain
The head and brain reflexes, which are located on the base and outside edges of the big toes and the thumb sides, will be treated.

Pituitary
The pituitary reflex is situated in the center of the fleshy part of the big toe, and it is found in a similar position on the thumb.

Solar plexus
The solar plexus reflex area is in zones 2 and 3 on the sole of the foot or the palm of the hand, just below the diaphragm level.

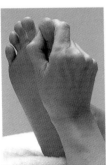
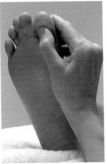
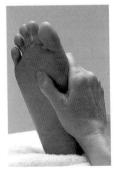

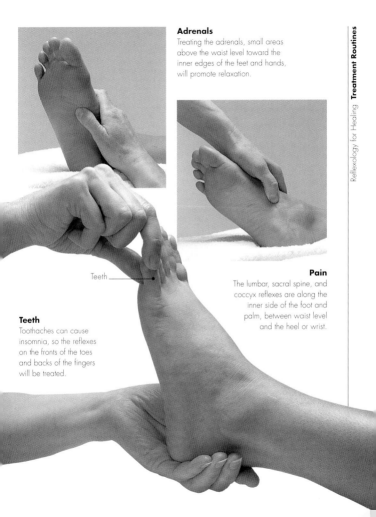

Adrenals
Treating the adrenals, small areas above the waist level toward the inner edges of the feet and hands, will promote relaxation.

Teeth

Pain
The lumbar, sacral spine, and coccyx reflexes are along the inner side of the foot and palm, between waist level and the heel or wrist.

Teeth
Toothaches can cause insomnia, so the reflexes on the fronts of the toes and backs of the fingers will be treated.

Back Problems

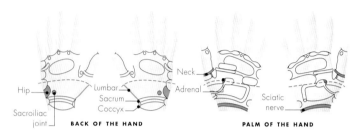

Hip

Sacroiliac joint

Lumbar
Sacrum
Coccyx

BACK OF THE HAND

Neck

Adrenal

Sciatic nerve

PALM OF THE HAND

Pain and stiffness in the back may be caused by disease, by injury to muscles or other soft tissues, a trapped nerve, and damage to joints or the disks between the spinal vertebrae. It is always wise to consult your doctor at the onset of back pain, but often it will be labeled "non-specific," which means that the cause is uncertain and the problem is likely to resolve itself. Although you can take some steps to reduce the chances of recurrence, once you have experienced back pain it is likely to recur at some stage. Osteopaths, chiropractors, and physical therapists can treat many back problems and this sort of treatment may help to avoid a recurrence.

Lower back pain

This can arise from problems in many areas of the body, apart from the spine itself, so treatment is likely to be given to reflexes for all the parts of the body that may be damaged or not working.

Sciatica

Inflammation of the sciatic nerve can cause excruciating pain in the lower back and buttocks and down into the thigh—in fact, anywhere along the path of this major nerve.

Treatment

Many back pain sufferers benefit from osteopathy or chiropractic treatment, especially when it is begun soon after the onset of pain. Reflexology treatment can also be very effective at relieving back pain, although this approach cannot pinpoint the actual cause of the problem. Treatment for back pain that results from an inflammatory condition such as rheumatoid arthritis or from the "bone thinning" disease osteoporosis can be effective, but should only be given by an experienced reflexologist.

Generally, the therapist will treat the spine and neck reflexes as part of a full treatment, but will also work on associated reflexes depending on the type and location of the pain. This may involve treating the adrenals when there is inflammation; the sciatic nerve and the various parts of the spine, including the coccyx, where there is injury or tension; and other joints, such as the hip or knee, if these appear to be involved.

Prevention

To prevent back problems, take care when lifting or moving heavy objects (including children) and get exercise to strengthen the back and stomach muscles and ligaments.

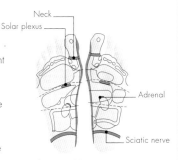

SOLE OF THE FOOT

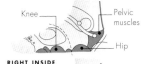

LEFT OUTSIDE

RIGHT INSIDE

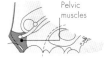

RIGHT OUTSIDE

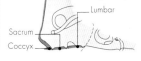

LEFT INSIDE

169

TREATMENT ROUTINES

For low back pain, the reflexologist will work all the spinal areas, from the cervical to the coccyx, as well as the neck itself. Other areas include the solar plexus (to ease pain and promote relaxation), the adrenals (for inflammation), and any parts of the body affected by referred pain or damage, such as the knees. The lumbar and sacral nerves in the lower back may need to be treated to ease sciatica.

Sciatic nerve
The sciatic nerve has a reflex area that runs in a band across the pad of the heel and the wrist.

Solar plexus
The solar plexus reflex is a small area on the sole, in Zones 2 and 3, just below the diaphragm line.

Coccyx
The coccyx reflex is just before the heel of the foot and the wrist, adjacent to the lumbar and sacrum reflexes.

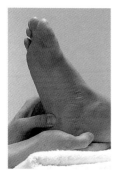

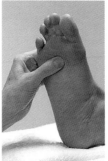

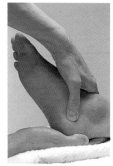

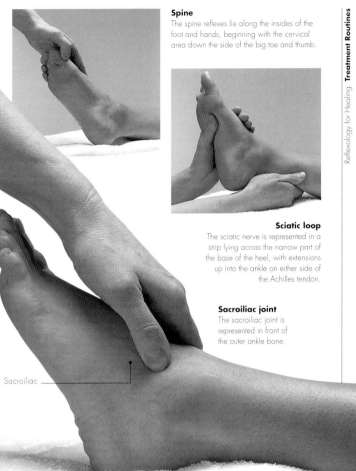

Spine

The spine reflexes lie along the insides of the foot and hands, beginning with the cervical area down the side of the big toe and thumb.

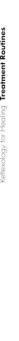

Sciatic loop

The sciatic nerve is represented in a strip lying across the narrow part of the base of the heel, with extensions up into the ankle on either side of the Achilles tendon.

Sacroiliac joint

The sacroiliac joint is represented in front of the outer ankle bone.

Sacroiliac

Muscle and Joint Pain

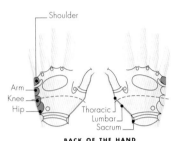

Shoulder

Arm
Knee
Hip
Thoracic
Lumbar
Sacrum

BACK OF THE HAND

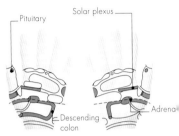

Pituitary

Solar plexus

Descending
colon

Adrenal

PALM OF THE HAND

Anyone who regularly takes part in a sport or who exercises strenuously is liable to suffer an injury at some point, and relatively unfit beginners are especially vulnerable. Strains and sprains are particularly common, and muscles and other soft tissue can easily be damaged by an awkward movement or a clumsy landing.

Reduce risk

It makes sense to minimize the risk by following a training program to build up strength and flexibility. You should always do warm-up and cool-down routines before and after a game or exercise session to protect your muscles. Treat an injury as soon as possible,

following what is called the RICE principle—Rest, Ice, Compression, and Elevation—but remember to wrap ice in fabric before applying it to your skin to prevent freezer burn.

RSI

Repetitive strain injury (RSI) is a type of overuse injury that can affect soft tissues in the shoulders, arms, and hands as a result of making the same movements repeatedly over a long period. This is usually job-related, and particularly affects keyboard workers and people who work on mechanized production lines. It is difficult to treat by orthodox methods, but reflexology can ease the pain and help the tissues to recover.

Arthritis

Arthritis can take many forms, all of which result in painful and inflamed joints. The most common form of joint disease is osteoarthritis, which most people develop to some degree as they get older. Osteoarthritis often affects joints which have been stressed by past sports activities: for example, professional soccer players may develop arthritis in their knee joints. In most cases, people with any kind of arthritis will be taking medication to suppress inflammation, ease the pain, and maintain mobility, and reflexology can help to increase its effectiveness.

The therapist will treat the particular areas of the body that are affected. The adrenals reflexes will also be treated if there is inflammation, and the solar plexus to encourage relaxation.

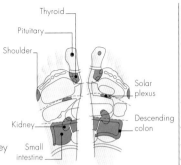

SOLE OF THE FOOT

Thyroid
Pituitary
Shoulder
Solar plexus
Kidney
Descending colon
Small intestine

LEFT OUTSIDE

Elbow
Hip
Knee

RIGHT INSIDE

Spine

RIGHT OUTSIDE

Arm
Shoulder

LEFT INSIDE

Spine

Self-help

Avoid putting unnecessary strain on joints by keeping your weight to a sensible level. Gentle exercise will strengthen the muscles that support the joints.

TREATMENT ROUTINES

The therapist will focus on the areas most badly affected. Rheumatoid arthritis sometimes affects the feet, and the reflexologist will need to work with great care, especially if damage to the joints means the hand cannot be treated instead. In cases of Repetitive Strain Injury (RSI), the affected areas or the zone-related area will be treated: the ankle for wrist pain, for example. The reflexes to be treated for sports injuries will depend on the site of the injury.

Hip

The hip reflex is on the outer side of the foot, within a small half-moon-shaped area just in front of the heel. It is between the wrist and waist level on the outer side of the back of the hands.

Arm

This reflex is located on the outer edge of the foot, running from the base of the little toe to the bony projection that is situated about halfway along the foot.

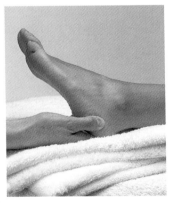

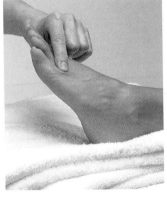

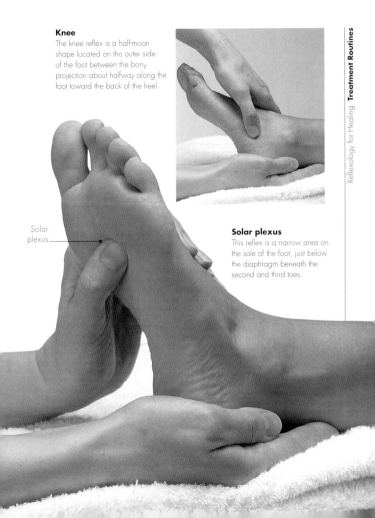

Knee

The knee reflex is a half-moon shape located on the outer side of the foot between the bony projection about halfway along the foot toward the back of the heel.

Solar plexus

Solar plexus

This reflex is a narrow area on the sole of the foot, just below the diaphragm beneath the second and third toes.

Eyes and Ears

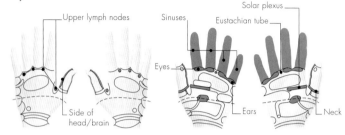

BACK OF THE HAND

Upper lymph nodes

Side of head/brain

PALM OF THE HAND

Solar plexus

Sinuses

Eustachian tube

Eyes

Ears

Neck

Anything other than minor and short-lived symptoms affecting the eyes or ears should be checked out by a doctor to rule out any potentially serious underlying condition. Deteriorating eyesight may sometimes be caused by a problem that requires conventional treatment and can develop as a result of damage to the back of the eye in people who are unaware that they have diabetes, for example. Gradual hearing impairment may not always be treatable, depending on the cause, but a doctor may recommend a hearing aid to improve the situation. Infection is a common cause of sore eyes and earaches. If the problem is persistent or the symptoms are more

than a nuisance it may sometimes be necessary to take antibiotics to eradicate it. Very often, however, problems with the eyes and ears are relatively insignificant in medical terms, but are nevertheless the source of considerable discomfort and disruption to normal activities.

Conjunctivitis

When the membrane lining the eyelid becomes inflamed—either as a result of infection or an allergic reaction—the eyes becomes red and itchy and sometimes sore. The condition is called conjunctivitis, and a reflexologist will treat the direct reflex area—for the eye —and associated reflex areas, such as the upper lymphatics if the symptoms are caused by an infection, the adrenals for an allergic reaction and, sometimes, the kidneys, which are zone-related—they are in the same longitudinal energy zone as the eyes.

Earaches and tinnitus

Earaches are often the result of an infection and the reflexologist will treat the direct reflex for the ear, the upper lymphatics to clear the infection, the Eustachian tubes to ease congestion, and the solar plexus for relaxation.

A ringing or buzzing in the ears can sometimes be associated with an ear infection—a distressing condition known as tinnitus. Orthodox medicine has little to offer by way of effective treatment, although some people find that electronic devices that emit "white noise" help to mask the sounds, and therapy may help a person to live with the symptoms more easily. In cases of tinnitus the reflexologist will also treat the side of the head, neck, cervical spine, and sinuses.

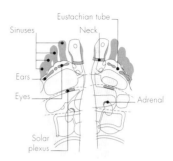

SOLE OF THE FOOT

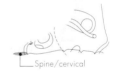

RIGHT INSIDE

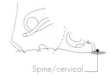

LEFT INSIDE

TREATMENT ROUTINES

For ear disorders, in addition to the ear reflex, the therapist will treat the Eustachian tube, which links the throat and the middle ear. If it becomes congested as a result of infection or an allergic reaction, it can affect the hearing and may sometimes cause tinnitus. When the eyes are sore due to a mild allergy or after a foreign body has been removed, irritation can be eased by treating the eye reflex area.

Earaches

The ear reflex is found along a narrow strip on the sole of the foot, below the base of the fourth and fifth toes. In the hand, it is in the palm, just below the point where the ring finger and little finger join the hand.

Congestion

The reflex area for the Eustachian tube is on the sole of the foot, just below the point where the third and fourth toes meet. On the hand, it is in the palm, just below the base of the third and fourth finger junction.

Alternative reflex

The Eustachian tube reflex may occasionally be found in similar positions located on the top of the foot and on the back of the hand. In this case it is situated above the junction between the third and fourth toes or fingers.

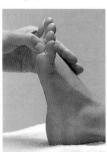
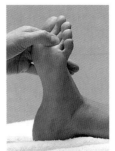
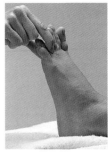

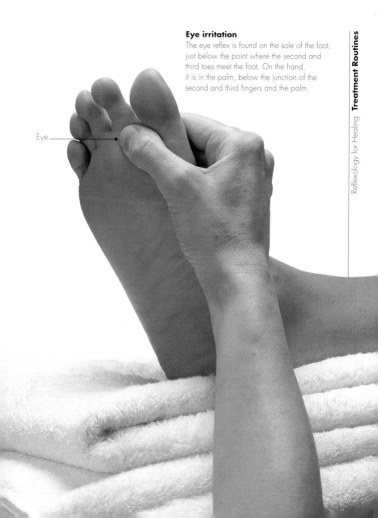

Eye irritation

The eye reflex is found on the sole of the foot, just below the point where the second and third toes meet the foot. On the hand, it is in the palm, below the junction of the second and third fingers and the palm.

Eye

Allergies

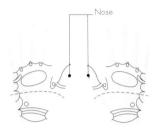

BACK OF THE HAND

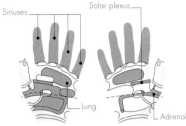

PALM OF THE HAND

An allergic reaction develops when the immune system reacts to the presence of a substance in the body that is actually harmless as though it were a virus, bacterium, or toxin of some kind. The offending substance, known as an allergen, may be swallowed, inhaled, come into contact with the skin, or enter the body through the skin—as with a bee sting. The immune system marshals its army of defenders, including histamines and other cells, to attack the "invader," and this can trigger a range of symptoms. Allergic reactions of this kind are becoming increasingly common, including potentially life-threatening ones such as asthma and peanut allergy.

Symptoms

Depending on the particular type of allergy, the result may be hay fever or rhinitis; a skin rash of some kind; respiratory symptoms such as asthma, nausea, and vomiting; or, just occasionally, a severe, life-threatening reaction that is known as anaphylaxis. The latter is an emergency that must be treated promptly with an injection of epinephrine.

It is important to try and identify what triggers the allergic reaction in any individual case, and to take as many steps as possible to avoid or minimize contact with the specific allergen(s) responsible. Very often the culprit is easy to identify: many people with asthma are allergic to the droppings of the house-dust mite and/or animal dander, for example, and hay fever sufferers react to various pollens. People with asthma will need to take regular medication to prevent attacks and to treat them when they occur, and medication is also often needed to suppress the symptoms of other allergies.

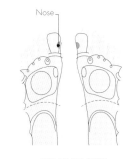

TOP OF THE FOOT

Reducing symptoms

Although no practitioner—whether orthodox or complementary—can claim to cure allergies, treatment may help to subdue the allergic reaction and so minimize symptoms. The reflexologist will attempt to do this by treating the reflex areas for the parts of the body affected by symptoms. Depending on the particular allergy, the direct reflexes may include the nose, sinuses, lungs, skin, and the digestive system. Treating the adrenals and the spleen may help to tone down the allergic response, and treatment of the solar plexus can help to encourage relaxation, which may be of particular benefit to people with asthma.

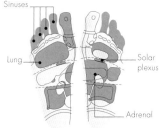

SOLE OF THE FOOT

TREATMENT ROUTINES
Depending on the specific allergy, many different parts of the body can be affected by symptoms, so the prime reflex areas to be treated will vary accordingly. In the case of asthma, for example, one important focus will be the lungs. Other significant areas might be the nose, eyes, sinuses, throat, and Eustachian tubes, and the adrenals and solar plexus will be treated in all allergic conditions to ease symptoms and promote relaxation.

Lungs
This reflex is represented on the sole of the foot, across almost the whole width of the ball beneath the second to the fifth toes. On the hand, the lung reflex is situated in the area of the palm immediately below the bases of the four fingers.

Sinuses
The sinus reflexes are on the base and sides of the toes and the front and sides of the fingers. It is important to treat the sinuses thoroughly in anyone who has an allergy such as hay fever or perennial rhinitis, which cause excess mucus and/or congestion.

Adrenals
The adrenal reflexes are small areas located just above waist level on the soles and palms, toward the inner edges of the feet and hands. Treating the adrenals will help to ease pain such as headaches that result from an allergic response.

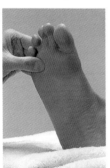
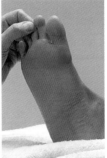
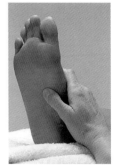

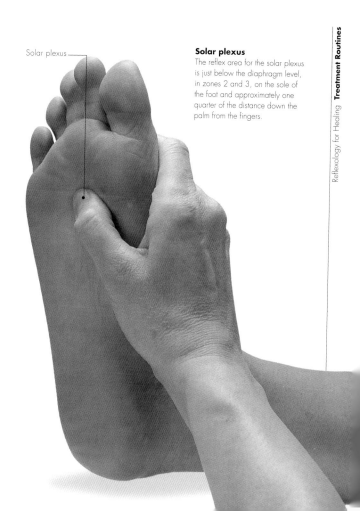

Solar plexus

Solar plexus

The reflex area for the solar plexus is just below the diaphragm level, in zones 2 and 3, on the sole of the foot and approximately one quarter of the distance down the palm from the fingers.

Following Up

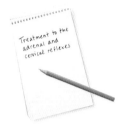

Note-taking
The reflexologist will make a record of the patient's treatment.

Before the course of treatment begins, the reflexologist will discuss how many treatments are likely to be needed. Each session normally lasts an hour, and in most cases, a minimum of three sessions will be needed before it is possible to assess whether the patient is deriving any real benefit. The length of the complete course will vary, but an average course will consist of around three to six sessions given once a week. There is rarely any point in continuing to have further sessions after that if there has been no improvement by that stage.

Aftereffects

The rate and type of response to treatment are a very individual matter. Many people will experience immediate aftereffects within a day or so of treatment—for example, they may find they need to pass urine or move their bowels more often than usual, or they may develop slight nausea, a short-lived headache, or a skin rash. All of these are signs that the body is responding actively to treatment and beginning to heal itself. Complementary therapists refer to this as a "healing crisis," thought to indicate the removal of "toxins" which have been stirred up by treatment.

Timescale

Where treatment has been given for a specific condition or symptoms, it is likely to be some time before any major improvement is experienced as the original energy imbalances gradually correct themselves. Sometimes, although the treatment may not have any very noticeable effect on their symptoms, the person being treated may find that their sense of overall well-being improves and they are better able to tolerate the symptoms than before.

Record-keeping

Every reflexologist will keep a detailed record of each patient, summarizing the initial problems, symptoms, and other relevant information, noting exactly what treatment has been given in each session, the patient's response, and the outcome of the treatment. Once the course is complete, she may recommend a maintenance program of less frequent treatment sessions to help to sustain the benefits over the longer term.

Many people who feel they have benefited from reflexology continue to have a session at regular intervals, perhaps every four to six weeks or so, in order to sustain the improvement in their health and help them cope with the stresses of everyday life. Treatment can help them again in the future if they have a recurrence of an earlier problem or develop a new one.

REFLEXOLOGY FOR SPECIAL CASES

People of all ages can enjoy the benefits of reflexology, but there may be differences in the approach to treatment at particular stages in life. Special care and considerable experience are needed when treating a pregnant woman, and she should not consider treating herself without expert guidance. ❧ Babies and children often respond well to reflexology, but it is unrealistic to expect them to sit still patiently for a full hour of treatment, so each session is likely to be shorter than normal. ❧ Older people often enjoy the physical contact that is involved in reflexology, which can help to relieve minor as well as more serious ailments. ❧ For complete maps of all the reflex areas see pages 30–37.

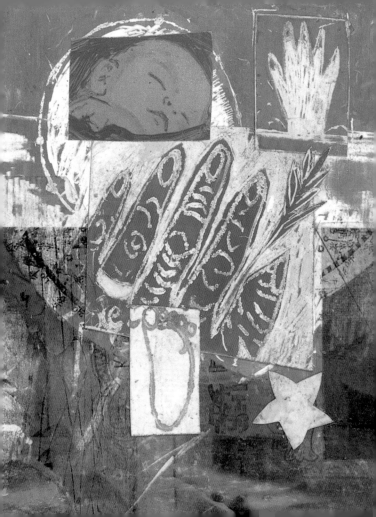

Babies and Children

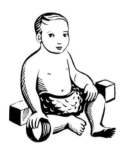

An early start
The young can derive as many benefits from reflexology as adults.

Seating

A baby or young child is likely to be more relaxed if she sits on her mother's lap during the treatment; the practitioner can then sit slightly to one side in order to work on her.

It is important to arrange things so that all three participants are feeling comfortable while the treatment is being done. An older child can sit in the reclining chair if she is tall enough to do so comfortably with her feet in an accessible position.

Treatment

The reflexologist may choose to treat either the hands or the feet, or both, depending on which area the child tolerates most easily.

In either case, the therapist must be even more precise than when treating adults because the reflex areas on a baby's or young child's foot or hand will be extremely small. Despite their size, however, treatment is carried out in pretty much the same way as it is conducted for an adult.

I n principle, giving reflexology to a baby or young child is the same as giving it to an adult, but in practice there are likely to be several differences in the way the therapist works. Obviously, most of the discussion about symptoms, diet, and so on will be between the therapist and the parent or other adult who has brought her for treatment, although an older child may want to discuss this with the therapist. Encourage children to be involved in their treatment in this way.

When to stop

Usually, a child will enjoy the treatment and a baby or toddler may even regard it as a kind of game, but if a young patient becomes distressed or restless, it is better to stop for a moment. She may be ready for some more treatment in a while, but there is no point in persisting if she is uncooperative.

Results

Children often respond more quickly than adults to reflexology, perhaps because their bodies have lost none of their innate ability to heal themselves. Their energy flow is more easily unblocked and the proper balance restored. Reflexology is often particularly beneficial for children who, while not actually very ill, have troublesome symptoms which are distressing them: teething pain, colic, and motion sickness, for example. It can also be helpful for treating emotional problems, such as anxiety, and for tackling chronic conditions such as asthma and other allergies.

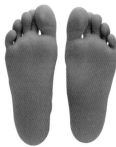

Treating children
Treatment should take around 30 minutes for a baby or toddler, about half the time of treating an adult, because the reflex areas are so much smaller.

THE RIGHT APPROACH

When a young child is being given reflexology treatment, the therapist and the child's parent need to work together. It is a question of finding the best means of keeping the child comfortable and relatively still long enough to enable the reflexologist to do her job, yet not continuing for so long that the child becomes distressed.

Childhood ailments
School-age children tend to get frequent bumps and bruises while playing and are also prone to minor viral infections, such as colds and tonsillitis, plus a condition known as "glue ear," when the middle ear becomes blocked with mucus.

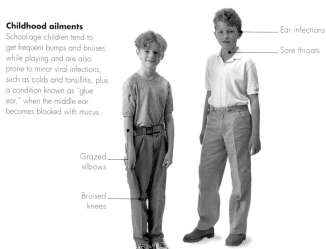

Ear infections

Sore throats

Grazed elbows

Bruised knees

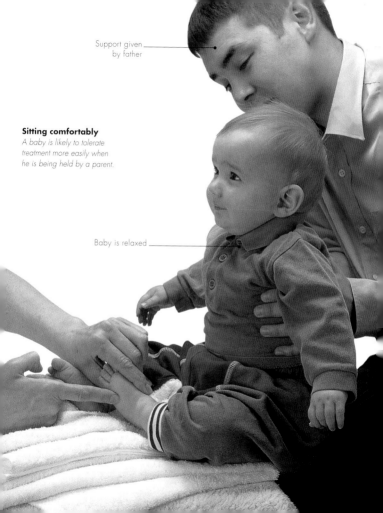

Support given by father

Sitting comfortably
A baby is likely to tolerate treatment more easily when he is being held by a parent.

Baby is relaxed

Babies' Problems

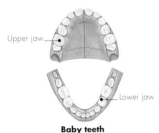

Upper jaw

Lower jaw

Baby teeth
*Children's milk teeth begin
to emerge from the age
of six months.*

I t is very distressing for parents when their baby is clearly in pain and crying, even though they have done everything they can think of to make her comfortable and contented.

Colic

One of the most common reasons for severe distress in the first three months of a baby's life is colic. The baby screams as if in agony, brings her knees up to her chest, and often turns red in the face. These bouts often occur at the same time each day, mostly in the early evening, and can last for several hours.

No one is really sure what causes the problem, although it probably has something to do with the immaturity of the newborn's nervous system, and most babies stop having the attacks around three months or so after they are born. A reflexologist may be able to ease the symptoms with a course of treatment, which will include working the reflex area for the intestines.

Teething

This can produce a number of troublesome symptoms, including pain, poor appetite, and sleeplessness. Reflexology can help to soothe a distressed baby and ease the pain.

Eczema

This distressing skin condition—which causes redness, itchiness, and flaking—is common in babies, especially in areas where the skin is dry and in skin creases. Symptoms may be eased by moisturizing creams and soap substitutes, and reflexology may alleviate the condition.

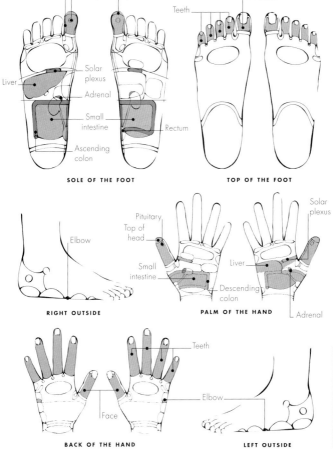

SOLE OF THE FOOT

Side of head
Pituitary
Top of head
Liver
Solar plexus
Adrenal
Small intestine
Rectum
Ascending colon

TOP OF THE FOOT

Teeth
Face

RIGHT OUTSIDE

Elbow

PALM OF THE HAND

Pituitary
Top of head
Small intestine
Solar plexus
Liver
Descending colon
Adrenal

BACK OF THE HAND

Teeth
Face

LEFT OUTSIDE

Elbow

SPECIAL ROUTINES FOR BABIES

To treat a baby with colic, the reflex area for the large intestine (on the sole of the foot, comprising several distinct elements) will be addressed. Treatment for teething will focus on the teeth and gum reflexes, found on the front of the toes. Treatment for eczema will be concentrated on the part of the body affected (and the adrenal glands, to reduce inflammation, allergies, and stress).

Colic—colon

The ascending colon, in zones 4 and 5 of the right foot, is from just above the pad of the heel up to the waist level; and the transverse colon crosses both feet at waist level. In the left foot, it turns through a right angle again and the descending colon extends down the left foot to a point just above the pad of the heel. The reflex for the sigmoid colon runs from here across all zones, where it meets the reflex for the rectum on the inner edge of the foot.

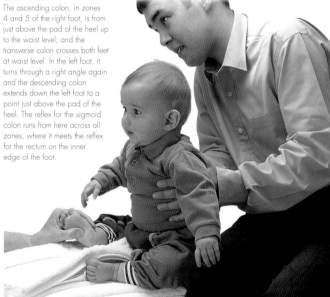

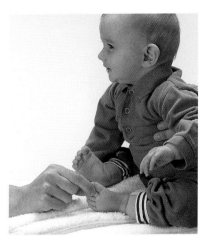

Teething pain—teeth

The reflexes for the teeth and gums are found on the front of the toes, just below the nails, with the front teeth in zones 1 and 2, and working across to the back teeth in zone 4. (In adults, the wisdom teeth reflexes are in zone 5.)

Eczema—face, elbows, and knees

Treatment for eczema is concentrated on the areas of skin most affected with scaliness and itching: commonly the face, elbows, and knees. The face reflexes are on the front of the big toes, below the nails; the elbow and knee reflex areas are found on the outer side of the foot, just behind the heel.

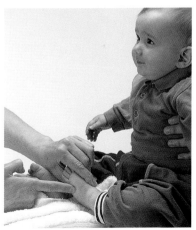

Problems of Older Children

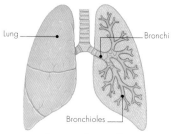

Lung

Bronchi

Bronchioles

Lungs under attack
*Today, allergic conditions
such as asthma are
increasing.*

Psychological and emotional
problems often manifest themselves
as physical symptoms, including
digestive complaints, difficulty sleeping,
and increased susceptibility to colds
and other infections. Reflexology is well
suited to treating symptoms in children
of this age, especially when stress and
anxiety are affecting their health.

Asthma
A child with asthma will need to be
on regular medication under the
supervision of a doctor, but reflexology

treatment of the direct reflexes, including
the lungs and bronchi, may help to
ease airway constriction; associated
reflexes may encompass the solar
plexus and diaphragm for relaxation;
the adrenals to reduce stress and
weaken the allergic response; and the
cervical and thoracic spine to improve
nerve supply to the lungs and bronchi.

Anxiety and stress
Treatment of the whole body through the
feet with emphasis on the solar plexus
and adrenals will help adolescents
suffering from anxiety or stress. Treating
the pituitary reflex will also help to
encourage hormone balance and
so ease symptoms arising from the
hormonal surges that begin at puberty.

Motion sickness
Treating the reflex areas for the ears can
ease symptoms because the inner ear
is important in maintaining balance
and creating awareness of the body's
movement and position in relation to
the external environment.

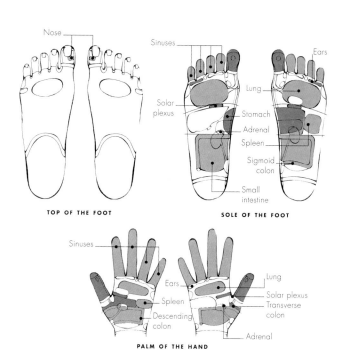

TOP OF THE FOOT

Nose

SOLE OF THE FOOT

Sinuses
Ears
Lung
Solar plexus
Stomach
Adrenal
Spleen
Sigmoid colon
Small intestine

PALM OF THE HAND

Sinuses
Ears
Lung
Solar plexus
Transverse colon
Spleen
Descending colon
Adrenal

BACK OF THE HAND

Nose

OLDER CHILDREN

Here are some special routines for older children. The main reflexes to be treated for asthma are those for the lungs and bronchi. In asthma as well as in other allergic conditions, treating the reflexes for the adrenals may help to tone down the abnormal immune system response. A course of reflexology—treating the solar plexus reflex area in particular—may relieve anxiety and encourage relaxation. The reflex areas for the ears will be treated to ease symptoms of travel sickness.

Asthma—lungs

The lung reflex is positioned on the ball of the foot, below the second to fifth toes. In the hands, the lung reflex lies below the fingers in the palm of the hand.

Motion sickness—ear reflexes

The ear reflexes are found just below where the fourth and fifth toes join the sole of the foot, and in the hand in the palm just below the junction with the fourth and fifth fingers.

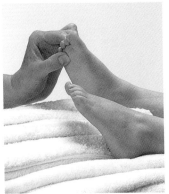

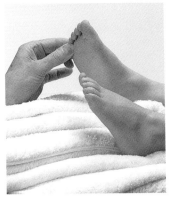

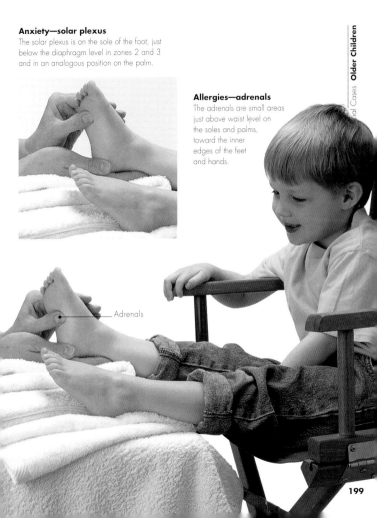

Anxiety—solar plexus

The solar plexus is on the sole of the foot, just below the diaphragm level in zones 2 and 3 and in an analogous position on the palm.

Allergies—adrenals

The adrenals are small areas just above waist level on the soles and palms, toward the inner edges of the feet and hands.

Adrenals

Pregnant Women

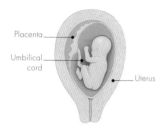

A new life
The body undergoes enormous changes during pregnancy.

Placenta

Umbilical cord

Uterus

Reflexology can be very effective in alleviating many troublesome ailments in pregnancy, but it is essential that the treatment is given by an experienced reflexologist. Self-treatment is generally not advised.

Contraindications

Generally, practitioners avoid treating a woman during the first trimester, especially if this is her first pregnancy, or if she has a history of miscarriage. These restrictions may not always apply if the woman has been having regular reflexology treatment before conceiving.

Morning sickness

Nausea and sickness usually disappear toward the end of the first trimester, but can be extremely debilitating. If an experienced reflexologist judges that it is safe to treat during this period, working the reflex area for the stomach may relieve the symptoms, and may also help the minority whose nausea continues beyond the first three months.

Emotional problems

The benefits of reflexology go beyond easing physical symptoms. Many women find they get very tired and stressed. This can contribute to emotional swings which are partly hormone-related but which may also reflect doubts and worries about the pregnancy itself. Regular sessions with a reflexologist can help with this process of adjustment and, as well as the benefits of the treatment itself, give the woman an opportunity to take a brief "time out" and come to terms with what is happening to her emotionally, psychologically, and physically.

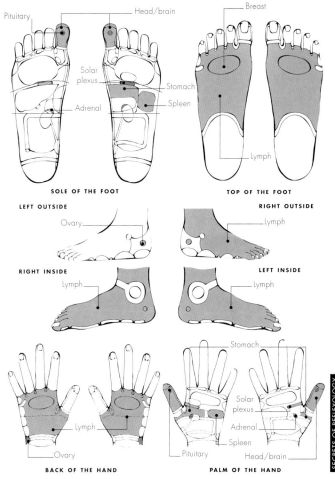

SOLE OF THE FOOT

Pituitary

Head/brain

Solar plexus

Stomach

Adrenal

Spleen

TOP OF THE FOOT

Breast

Lymph

LEFT OUTSIDE

RIGHT OUTSIDE

Ovary

Lymph

RIGHT INSIDE

LEFT INSIDE

Lymph

Lymph

BACK OF THE HAND

Lymph

Ovary

PALM OF THE HAND

Stomach

Solar plexus

Adrenal

Spleen

Pituitary

Head/brain

EARLY PREGNANCY

Any form of treatment or medication is generally not advised during the first three months of pregnancy, because this a critical stage in fetal development where things can easily go wrong. However, if an experienced reflexologist judges that it is safe to treat during this period, she may work on the areas for nausea, tiredness, and emotional problems. If you have never had reflexology before, consult your doctor before embarking upon treatment.

Nausea—stomach

This is treated with the stomach reflex, which is primarily in the sole of the foot, in zones 1 to 3 between the waist and diaphragm levels. It is represented in comparable regions of the palms of both hands.

Tiredness—spleen

This a common problem arising from the increased demands on the woman's body. Treatment will be focused on the spleen reflex. This is found on the sole of the left foot and the palm of the left hand, in zones 4 and 5 between the waist and diaphragm levels.

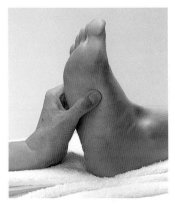

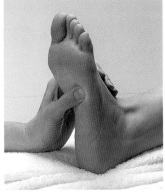

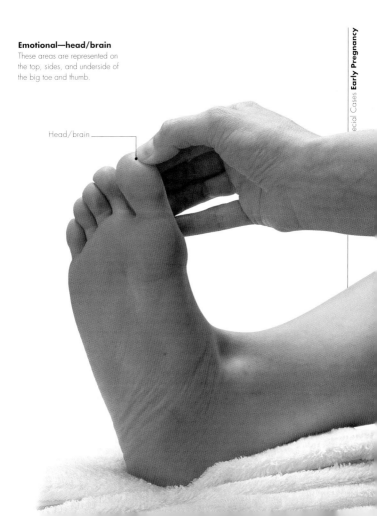

Emotional—head/brain
These areas are represented on
the top, sides, and underside of
the big toe and thumb.

Head/brain

Special Routines for Later Pregnancy

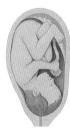

Problems

The increasing size and weight of the uterus can trigger problems.

Pain in the lower back is common as the woman unconsciously adjusts her posture by swaying back to balance the weight of the baby. This stress is exacerbated by the effect of pregnancy hormones, which relax the ligaments holding the sacro-iliac joint firmly in place so as to allow the pelvis to expand and allow the baby to pass into the birth canal.

Varicose veins may develop in the lower legs and around the anus (hemorrhoids, or piles) as a result of changes caused by the expanding uterus and the actions of hormones. The passage of the contents of the bowels can be slowed, causing constipation.

Lack of sleep is often a problem toward the end of pregnancy, when it can be almost impossible to find a comfortable position. Any worries or anxiety about the imminent birth can make it even harder to sleep.

Treatment

Reflexology can help not only by treating specific symptoms, but also by encouraging relaxation and restoring the body's natural energy balance. In addition to giving a whole body treatment, extra attention will be given to the direct reflex areas related to any symptoms. These might include the lower spine for back pain, the intestines for constipation, the rectum and anus for hemorrhoids, the kidneys for swollen ankles caused by fluid retention, and the head and brain for insomnia.

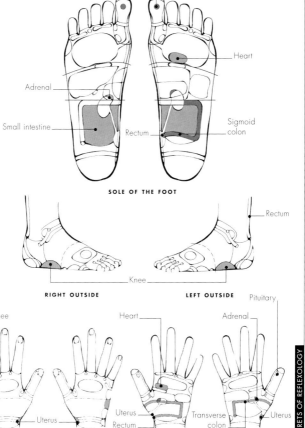

Pituitary

Heart

Adrenal

Small intestine

Rectum

Sigmoid colon

SOLE OF THE FOOT

Rectum

Knee

RIGHT OUTSIDE

LEFT OUTSIDE

Pituitary

Knee

Heart

Adrenal

Uterus

Uterus

Rectum

Transverse colon

Uterus

BACK OF THE HAND

PALM OF THE HAND

LATER PREGNANCY

Treating the lumbar and sacral spine reflexes will help to ease back pain caused by poor posture and the joint-loosening effects of pregnancy hormones. Treatment may also ease the discomfort of varicose veins and may prevent the problem from worsening. The overall balancing effect of a course of reflexology may ease sleep problems, and the therapist will pay extra attention to the pituitary gland, which controls and regulates hormone production throughout the body.

Backache—spine

Lumbar and sacral spine reflexes are found on the inner side of the foot, starting at the waist level and extending to the coccyx, just in front of the heel. On the hand, the lower spine is represented along the edge from the base of the thumb to just before the wrist.

Hemorrhoids—rectum

The two zones to be treated are the rectum/anus, consisting of a narrow strip running up the back of the ankle, above the heel, and the area in zone 1 on the inner sole just above the heel pad, and on the hand below the thumb, just above the wrist.

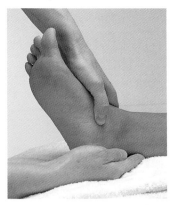

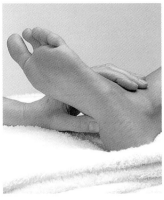

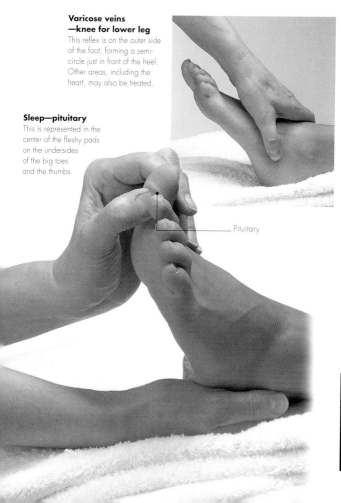

**Varicose veins
—knee for lower leg**

This reflex is on the outer side of the foot, forming a semi-circle just in front of the heel. Other areas, including the heart, may also be treated.

Sleep—pituitary

This is represented in the center of the fleshy pads on the undersides of the big toes and the thumbs.

Pituitary

Older People

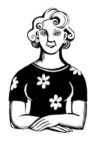

Beating isolation
Older clients may appreciate a therapist's counseling skills.

Getting older does not necessarily mean declining health, and many people remain fit and well in their later years, even though they may have less energy and suppleness than they once did. Nevertheless, some loss of muscle and skin tone is inevitable, and conditions such as osteoarthritis, cardiovascular disease, and deteriorating hearing and eyesight are more prevalent.

Unfortunately, loneliness and social isolation complicate the problems of failing health for some older people. It is also very easy to slip into the habit of eating a nutritionally poor diet, perhaps because it does not seem worth the effort of preparing and cooking proper meals when you're on your own. Many older people complain that they sleep less well than they did when younger, although this may be in part related to leading a less active life.

Social contact

Regular sessions with a concerned and sympathetic professional can offer much-needed social contact for older people. Some reflexologists develop a skill in counseling—someone who is alone a lot may appreciate the opportunity to air any emotional difficulties, although some will need encouragement to do so if they are unaccustomed to talking about their feelings. It may also take time for the person to relax sufficiently to enjoy the physical contact, although most people come to appreciate its benefits once they get used to the idea. Where appropriate, a therapist may be in a position to encourage a patient to seek

other kinds of expert help—whether
from their doctor or from another health
professional, such as a podiatrist,
for example.

Treatment

A combination of factors may well result
in energy blockages or imbalances,
and reflexology can bring about an
improvement in a person's overall sense
of well-being by restoring this balance
through a course of treatment. If some
reflex areas are unusually tender, this
will indicate to the reflexologist that
certain parts of the body are not
working as well as they should because
of energy imbalances and blockages.
A course of treatment can help to tone
up the body's systems, increasing
energy levels and resistance to illness,
as well as treating specific symptoms.

Arthritis

For more detailed information about
reflexology and other treatments for arthritis
see pages 172–175.

PRACTICAL TIPS

Before beginning a course of treatment for an older person, the reflexologist will take time to make sure she is comfortable and able to relax in the treatment chair. She may also offer advice on caring for the skin, which may be dry and delicate, and for the feet. An older person may need treatment from a podiatrist for hard skin and to have her toenails cut if she finds this difficult to do herself.

Arthritis—hips

Some degree of arthritis in the joints, especially the hips and knees, is almost universal and may require special treatment (see page 173). The hip reflex is on the outside of the foot just in front of the heel.

Arthritis—hands

If the joints in the hands are swollen and/or painful, then the zone-related reflexes in the feet, such as the top of the feet, may be treated instead.

Psychological problems —head/brain

Emotional and psychological problems may be eased by treatment to the head zones, on the top of the big toe above the nail and down the inner side of the big toe.

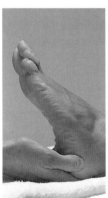
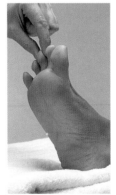
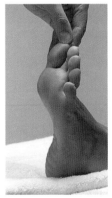

Bladder control—bladder
Difficulties with bladder control must be handled with great tact, but treating the bladder reflex may help to ease the symptoms.

Cutting the toenails
If an older person is unable to trim her own toenails, the reflexologist may do it, if she cannot get to see a podiatrist.

Cut is made straight across

Special Routines for Older People

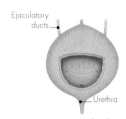

Ejaculatory ducts

Urethra

Prostate gland

Milky fluid is combined with seminal fluid in this gland.

The prostate is a small gland that lies between the bladder and the base of the penis and often causes problems in older men, usually after the age of about 60. It may become enlarged, eventually compressing the urethra and sometimes the bladder, causing problems with urination, and in some instances may become cancerous. As part of treatment of the whole body to restore harmony and energy balance, and improve the man's sense of well-being, the therapist will pay particular attention to the prostate reflex.

Aftereffects of a stroke

When the blood supply to a part of the brain is interrupted, either because of a clot or a burst artery, the consequences depend on the severity of the damage and where it occurs. Possible problems include paralysis, visual disturbances, and communication and psychological difficulties. Reflex areas around the big toe and thumb, which represent the head and brain, will be treated.

Hearing and sight

Problems with hearing or sight will require special attention to the reflex areas for the ears and eyes. There is no cure for hearing loss that results simply from aging, but reflexology may help to slow any natural deterioration and treat problems which may be affecting the hearing, such as phlegm. By encouraging and maintaining a healthy flow of energy, reflexology can help to keep the eyesight as sharp as possible and may prevent it from getting worse.

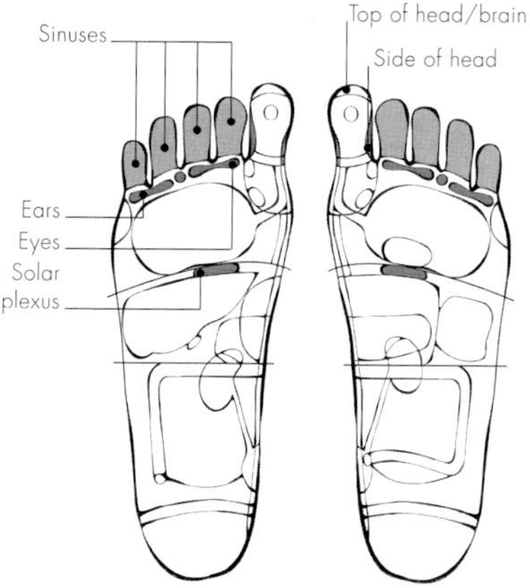

Sinuses

Top of head/brain

Side of head

Ears
Eyes
Solar
plexus

SOLE OF THE FOOT

RIGHT INSIDE

LEFT INSIDE

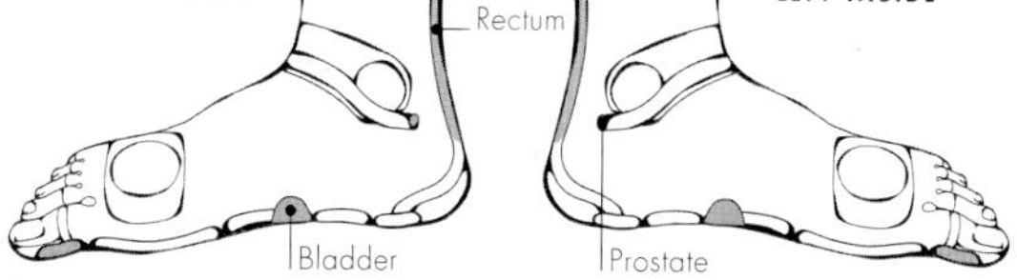

Rectum

Bladder

Prostate

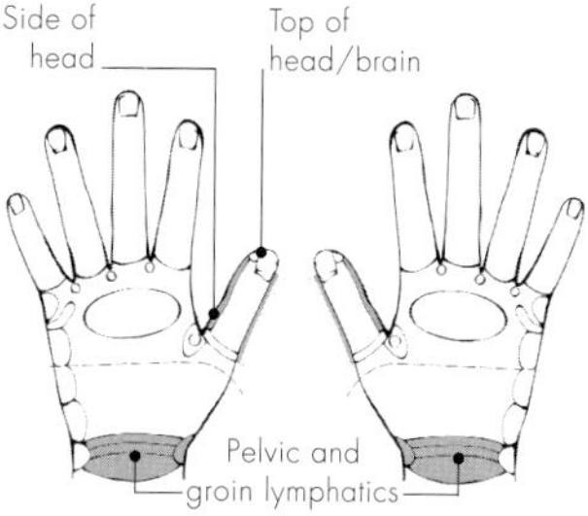

Side of
head

Top of
head/brain

Sinuses

Eyes

Ears

Kidney

Ureter

Pelvic and
groin lymphatics

Bladder

BACK OF THE HAND

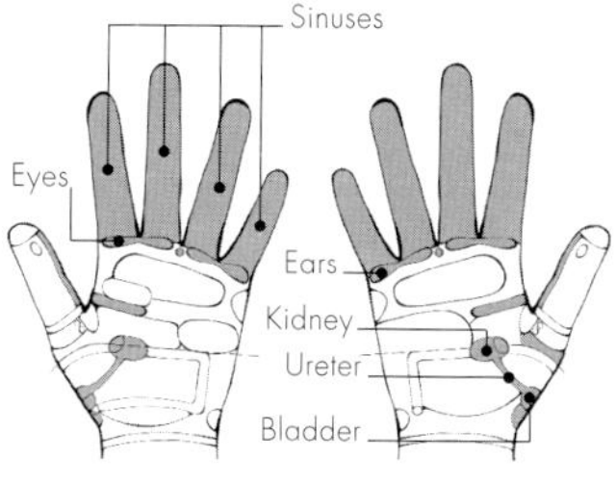

PALM OF THE HAND

TREATMENT

A course of reflexology may help to slow any natural deterioration in hearing and eyesight and treat problems, such as phlegm. The appropriate reflex point will be treated to minimize prostate problems, and in cases of stroke reflexology will aim to restore a natural energy balance to enable the person to make the best possible use of those functions unaffected by the damage to certain parts of the brain.

Ears

The ear reflexes are just below where the fourth and fifth toes join the sole of the foot, and to one side of the palm, below the junction with the fourth and fifth fingers.

Eyes

The eye reflex areas are on the sole of the foot, just under the junction with the second and third toes. Treatment may help to keep the eyesight as acute as possible.

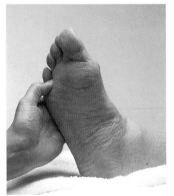

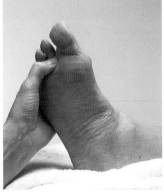

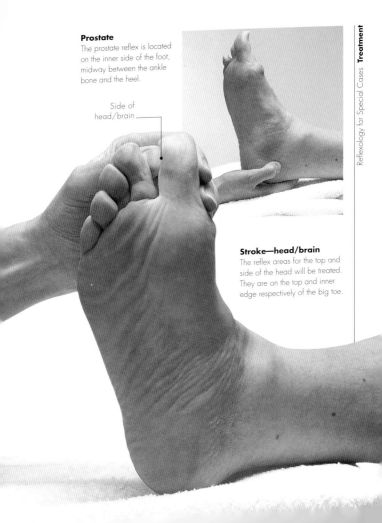

Prostate
The prostate reflex is located on the inner side of the foot, midway between the ankle bone and the heel.

Side of head/brain

Stroke—head/brain
The reflex areas for the top and side of the head will be treated. They are on the top and inner edge respectively of the big toe.

FURTHER READING

ARNOT, MICHELLE, *Foot Notes*, Sphere Books

BAYLY, DOREEN, *Reflexology Today*, Healing Arts Press

BYERS, DWIGHT C. *Better Health with Foot Reflexology*, Ingham Publishing

CHOPRA, DEEPAK, *Perfect Health*, Bantam Books

DOUGANS, INGE, *The Complete Illustrated Guide to Reflexology*, Element Books

DOUGANS, INGE WITH ELLIS, SUZANNE, *Reflexology: Foot Massage for Total Health*, Element Books

FAST, JULIUS, *You and Your Feet*, Pelham Books

FITZGERALD, WILLIAM H. AND BOWERS, EDWIN F., *Zone Therapy*, Health Research

GILLANDERS, ANN, *Reflexology—The Ancient Answer to Modern Ailments*, Gaia Books

GILLANDERS, ANN, *Reflexology: A Step-by-Step Guide*, Gaia Books

GOOSMAN-LEGGER, ASTRID, *Zone Therapy Using Foot Massage*, The C.W. Daniel Company Ltd.

GORE, ANYA, *Reflexology*, Optima

GRINBERG, AVI, *Holistic Reflexology*, Thorsons

HALL, NICOLA, *Reflexology— A Patient's Guide*, Thorsons

HALL, NICOLA, *Reflexology—A Way to Better Health*, Newleaf

INGHAM, EUNICE D., *Stories the Feet Can Tell Thru Reflexology*, Ingham Publishing

INGHAM, EUNICE D., *Stories the Feet Have Told Thru Reflexology*, Ingham Publishing

ISSEL, CHRISTINE, *Reflexology: Art, Science and History*, New Frontier Publishing

KUNZ, KEVIN AND BARBARA, *The Complete Guide to Foot Reflexology*, Thorsons

MARQUARDT, HANNE, *Reflex Zone Therapy of the Feet*, Healing Arts Press

NORMAN, LAURA, *Feet First*, Simon & Schuster

RUSSEL, LEWIS AND HARDY, BOB, *Healthy Feet*, Optima

STORMER, CHRIS, *Language of the Feet*, Hodder & Stoughton

STORMER, CHRIS, *Reflexology: The Definitive Guide*, Hodder & Stoughton

WAGNER, FRANZ, *Reflex Zone Massage*, Thorsons

USEFUL ADDRESSES

US AND CANADA

Foot Reflex Awareness Association
PO Box 7622, Mission Hills,
CA 91346

International Council of Reflexologists
PO Box 30513,
Richmond Hill,
Ontario L4C 0C7, Canada
(Fax: (905) 884 0294)

International Institute of Reflexology
PO Box 12642,
Saint Petersburg,
FL 33733
(Tel: (813) 343 4811)

Reflexology Assocation of America
4012 S. Rainbow Boulevard,
Box K585, Las Vegas,
NV 89103-2509

Reflexology Association of Canada (RAC)
11 Glen Cameron Road,
Unit 4, Thornhill,
Ontario L8T 4NB, Canada
(Tel: (905) 889 5900)

AUSTRALIA/NEW ZEALAND

Australian School of Reflexology
15 Kedumba Crescent,
Turramurra 2074,
New South Wales,
Australia
(Tel: (61) 299 883881)

New Zealand Institute of Reflexologists Inc.
39a Awarua Crescent,
Oraker, Auckland,
(Tel: (09) 522 6903)

Reflexology Association of Australia
PO Box 366,
Cammeray, New South Wales 2062,
(Tel: 0412 190 495)

UK AND IRELAND

Association of Reflexologists
27 Old Gloucester Street,
London WC1N 3XX, UK
(Tel: (0870) 567 3320)

Bayly School of Reflexology and British Reflexology Association
Monks Orchard,
Whitbourne,
Worcestershire WR6 5RB,
UK
(Tel: (01886) 821207)

British School of

Reflexology and Holistic Association of Reflexologists
92 Sheering Road,
Old Harlow,
Essex CM17 0JW, UK
(Tel: (01279) 429060)

International Federation of Reflexologists
76–8 Edridge Road,
Croydon, Surrey CR0 1EF, UK
(Tel: (0208) 667 9458)

Irish Reflexologists Institute
3 Blackglen Court,
Lambs Cross, Sandyford,
Dublin, Republic of Ireland

Scottish Institute of Reflexology
(Secretary: Ruth Marozzo)
4 Eden Road, Ednan, Kelso,
Roxburghshire TD5 7QG, UK
(Tel: (01573) 226645)

GLOSSARY

Acupuncture an ancient Chinese form of therapy that uses needles applied to specific points in the body to rebalance energy; some reflexologists believe that it works in a similar way to reflexology, although it uses different energy channels

Closing down the final stage of a treatment session, the purpose of which is to leave the individual feeling relaxed

Complementary therapy natural treatments that avoid the use of pharmaceutical drugs or surgery and are intended to "complement" rather than replace any orthodox treatment; practitioners follow a holistic approach rather than focusing on specific symptoms or conditions

Crystals small "gritty" areas under the skin of the feet or hands that may be tender to the touch; a sensitive reflexologist will become aware of them while working on an individual's feet and will regard them as an indication that there may be problems in the part of the body relating to the site of the crystal deposit

Diaphragm level an area between a "notional" line that crosses the foot just below the ball of the foot and the waist line; it is unrelated to the skeletal structure of the foot or hand, and is used to help practitioners pinpoint the position of reflex zones on the feet and hands with greater accuracy

Energy the energy flowing through the body along the longitudinal zones, which is rebalanced and unblocked by massaging the related reflex areas located in the hands and feet

Energy block a blockage in the flow of energy in one part of the body that will affect other structures lying in the same longitudinal zone and will need to be cleared by treating the reflex areas in the feet or hands within that zone

Energy imbalance when one part of the body is not working properly, energy will not be able to flow as it should through the longitudinal zones and the person concerned is likely to feel the ill effects of this imbalance; it may manifest itself in physical or psychological symptoms or simply as a general lack of well-being

Healing complementary therapists believe that the human body has the ability to heal itself naturally, and the purpose of treatment is to encourage this and so restore the individual to good health; it is more a question of tackling the underlying problem than of alleviating the symptoms

Holistic the holistic approach is the basis of all complementary therapies and simply means treating the whole person rather than concentrating on their disease or symptoms; thus therapists will be interested in every aspect of a patient's life, including their emotional concerns and anxieties, as well as their specific health problems, because these cannot be tackled in isolation

Kirlian photography a method of specialized photography developed in the former USSR, which uses high-voltage electricity to allow the levels of energy in the hands and feet to be visualized in the resulting "photograph"

Kneading using both hands to press on the top and bottom of the foot or hand in a rotating movement in order to aid relaxation

Longitudinal zones the ten "channels," five on either side of the body, extending from the tips of the toes to the head; it is through these zones that the vital energy flows, and points along the length of each zone are accessed on the hands and feet during treatment

Meridians the 14 channels of energy that are used by practitioners of acupuncture, which connect the interior parts of the body with the exterior

Overtreatment where an individual has symptoms suggesting that a particular part of the body is not working properly, the reflexologist will spend extra time treating the relevant reflex areas; however, it is necessary to find the right balance between giving sufficient treatment and overdoing it, causing undesirable side effects

Pelvic floor line a line visualized by reflexologists as passing horizontally across the foot over the tarsal bones of the heel between the ankle bones

Pituitary gland an important gland situated at the base of the brain, which plays a major role in controlling the interplay of hormones in the body

Recliner chair most reflexologists will have a special chair in their treatment room, which is designed to allow the recipient to relax comfortably during a session, with their legs slightly raised to enable the therapist to work on the feet without strain

Reflex areas these are shown on the maps of the hands and feet on pages 30–37; their position on the foot and hand reflects their position in the body

Self-treatment it is possible, though not easy, to treat some reflex areas on your own hands and feet; this is most appropriate to ease minor problems such as a headache, but cannot achieve the same beneficial effects as a full treatment from a therapist

Shoulder girdle a line visualized as lying across the foot at the level of the junction between the phalanges (the toe bones) and the metatarsal bones in the top part of the foot

Solar plexus breathing part of the "closing down" element of treatment; aids relaxation and promotes a feeling of calm in the person who is being treated

Transverse zones used as an aid to locating specific reflex areas, generally in the feet, and defined by a series of lines visualized as crossing the foot horizontally at several different points

Healing crisis this term is often used to describe the side effects that may be experienced by a patient following a session of reflexology treatment; although it may be an indication that the treatment is having the desired effect, it may also occasionally be a sign of overtreatment and should be reported to the therapist

Waist line a line that divides the foot horizontally at the level where the metatarsal bones in the top meet the first of the tarsal bones before the heel bones

Whole body treatment this refers to what happens in a reflexology treatment session—even where specific problems require extra attention to be devoted to particular reflexes, the whole of the feet (or hands) will be given treatment

Wringing holding the foot (or hand) in both hands, with one hand around the outer and one around the inner edge, then gently spreading the foot in order to move the bones apart from one another

Zone-related areas these give the therapist some alternatives if extra treatment is needed for an injury: for example, the knee might be massaged as additional therapy if the elbow were injured and could not be massaged directly

Zone therapy a therapy developed by American physician Dr. William Fitzgerald, who is regarded as a pioneer of modern reflexology; published in 1917, his book of the same name outlined the concept of energy flowing through ten longitudinal zones and how pressure treatment could unblock and rebalance this energy, with beneficial results for the patient

INDEX